Lei Chen
Editor

Women with Epilepsy in Child-bearing Age

Diagnosis and Treatment

Springer

Editor
Lei Chen
Department of Neurology
West China Hospital, Sichuan University
Chengdu, China

ISBN 978-981-97-3920-2 ISBN 978-981-97-3921-9 (eBook)
https://doi.org/10.1007/978-981-97-3921-9

This Springer imprint is published by the registered company Springer Nature Singapore Pte Ltd.
The registered company address is: 152 Beach Road, #21-01/04 Gateway East, Singapore 189721, Singapore

Foreword

Of the 70 million individuals living with epilepsy worldwide, at least 14 million are women of childbearing age. It is estimated that approximately 650,000 children are born to mothers diagnosed with epilepsy each year. While creating a family through childbirth is a significant life event, women with epilepsy in their childbearing years face unique challenges. Seizures and antiseizure medications can both impact sex hormones and fertility. Despite the teratogenic potential of some antiseizure medications, seizure prophylaxis during pregnancy is often necessary to prevent harm to both the mother and the fetus from uncontrolled seizures.

The difficulty that arises for both the patient and her physician is in striking a balance between the risks associated with seizures and those linked to treatment. This complexity is exacerbated by the influence of pregnancy on blood levels of antiseizure medications, requiring close monitoring and dose adjustments. The postpartum period also requires special attention to ensure safe breastfeeding and to prevent seizures triggered by sleep deprivation.

In the recent decades, significant progress has been made in the understanding and management of epilepsy in women of childbearing age, which has led to the development of evidence-based practices. However, the majority of the research conducted has originated from Western countries, despite the fact that the majority of the global population resides in other regions and particularly Asia. Due to variations in healthcare systems, resources, settings, and ethnicities, data from Western countries may not be directly applicable to other parts of the world such as China.

This book seeks to address this crucial knowledge gap by featuring expert authors from China who share their insights, research, and experiences in managing women with epilepsy. The content covers a spectrum of topics, from research findings to practical management recommendations, all within the Chinese context. While this book will be particularly valuable to practicing neurologists and epileptologists in China, it also holds relevance for those interested in cross-regional comparisons and the generalizability of observations and recommendations.

Introduction to Torbjörn Tomson

Torbjörn Tomson is Senior Professor of Neurology at the Department of Clinical Neuroscience, Karolinska Institutet, and Senior Consultant at the Department of

Neurology, Karolinska University Hospital, Stockholm, Sweden. His focus within the field of epilepsy research is on pharmacotherapy, epidemiology, and pregnancy issues. In addition, his main contributions to the field are in research on sudden unexpected death in epilepsy (SUDEP) as well as pregnancy outcomes in relation to the maternal use of different antiseizure medications. He has served on several commissions of the International League Against Epilepsy (ILAE) including the Task Force on Women and Pregnancy. Furthermore, he has been appointed Ambassador of Epilepsy by the ILAE and the International Bureau for Epilepsy, and in 2013, he received the America Epilepsy Society Research Recognition Award for Clinical Science.

Department of Clinical Neuroscience
Karolinska Institutet
Stockholm, Sweden

Torbjörn Tomson

Editorial Board

Contents

Disease Burden of Women with Epilepsy 1

Ding Ding, Leihao Sha, and Yiling Chen

1.1 The Uniqueness of Diagnosis and Treatment in Women with Epilepsy

Leihao Sha

Epilepsy is a chronic brain disorder characterized by recurrent, episodic, and transient central nervous system dysfunction caused by the abnormal excessive discharge of neurons in the brain. It is the second commonest central nervous system disorder. The risk of death for people with epilepsy is 2–3 times higher than that of the general population, with the main causes being sudden unexpected death in epilepsy (SUDEP), status epilepticus, accidental injury, and suicide. There are approximately 60 million people diagnosed with epilepsy worldwide, with a lifetime prevalence and annual incidence rate of 7.6/1000 and 67.77/100,000, respectively. The incidence rates are similar between males and females. According to statistics, the prevalence of epilepsy in women is about 6.85/1000, with approximately 40% of diagnosed women in their reproductive years. Epileptic seizures affect 0.3–0.7% of pregnant women with epilepsy (WWE).

As a special group of people with epilepsy, female patients have specific needs and concerns at every stage of life, from birth to adulthood and old age (Christian et al. 2020) (Fig. 1.1). The hormonal changes that occur throughout a woman's life can both affect and be affected by the mechanisms of seizure occurrence as well as antiseizure medications (ASMs), leading to fluctuations in ASM concentrations and changes in treatment efficacy. Sodium valproate is associated with the development of polycystic ovary syndrome in WWE, and this can affect reproductive endocrine

D. Ding (✉) · Y. Chen
Department of Neurology, Fudan University Huashan Hospital, Shanghai, China

L. Sha
Department of Neurology, West China Hospital, Sichuan University, Chengdu, China

L. Chen (ed.), *Women with Epilepsy in Child-bearing Age*,
https://doi.org/10.1007/978-981-97-3921-9_1

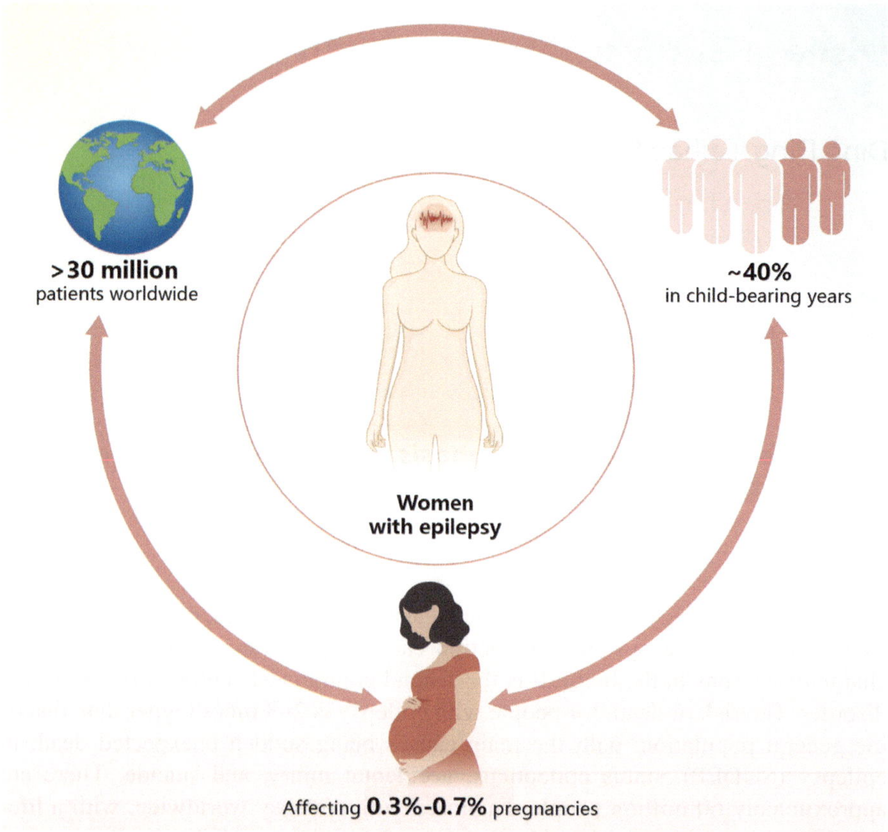

Fig. 1.1 Overview of WWE

function. Furthermore, epilepsy is the commonest neurological complication experienced during pregnancy, occurring in approximately 1% of pregnant women. Due to the increased obstetric and fetal complications observed in pregnant WWE, they are considered a high-risk group. WWE are at increased risk of miscarriage, stillbirth, preterm birth, preeclampsia, and early vaginal bleeding during pregnancy. Compared with healthy controls, the risk of maternal mortality during pregnancy in WWE is increased five- to tenfold. In addition, the offspring of people with epilepsy are at increased risk of severe congenital malformations and adverse neurological development compared with the general population. The proportion of major congenital malformations associated with different types of ASMs is 2–10%. The risk of developing neurodevelopmental disorders (including autism spectrum disorders, intellectual disabilities, and psychiatric disorders) is 2–5 times higher in the offspring of people with epilepsy compared to the offspring of healthy controls. Moreover, children born to WWE during pregnancy may also experience delayed or abnormal neurological development, including impairments in language cognitive skills and memory as well as behavioral abnormalities. The risk of postpartum depression in WWE is also several times higher than that in healthy pregnant women. These findings indicate that pregnant WWE and their children usually require dedicated medical care and treatment throughout the gestational period and beyond, which has profound medical and economic implications.

The above findings demonstrate that WWE experience a unique disease course, and management of their epilepsy is associated with specific challenges. Therefore, in order to provide targeted treatment plans and feedback for these individuals, there is a need to combine multiple aspects such as the diagnosis of seizure types and syndromes, the impact of sex hormones on epilepsy, and the impact of epilepsy and treatment on fertility.

This chapter aims to provide an overview on the current status of research relating to the overall management of female patients with epilepsy, in order to assist the scientific diagnosis, treatment, and efficient management of female patients with epilepsy.

1.2 Disease Burden and Quality of Life in Women with Epilepsy

Ding Ding and Yiling Chen

1.2.1 Epidemiological Data on Epilepsy Disease Burden by Sex

Epilepsy ranks as the second most prevalent neurological disorder, affecting roughly one in 26 individuals during their lifetime (GBD 2016 Epilepsy Collaborators 2019). The term "epilepsy" encompasses a spectrum of disorders marked by recurrent spontaneous seizures. It impacts individuals of all genders and ages throughout their lives. Presently, treatment primarily involves ASMs, tailored in type, quantity, and dosage to the patient's age and epilepsy form. For some, particularly children, dietary therapies complement ASMs. Regrettably, about one-third of epilepsy patients find current treatments ineffective. While surgical removal of the seizure-originating tissue is viable for certain patients, it remains impractical for others and may lead to negative side effects. Moreover, seizure relapses and their physical and psychological impacts render epilepsy a challenging neurological condition.

1.2.1.1 Global Prevalence, Morbidity, and Mortality of Epilepsy

A study published in Lancet Neurology provides a systematic description of the global burden of epilepsy between 2009 and 2016. In 2016, there were 45.9 million patients with all active epilepsy globally (both idiopathic and secondary epilepsy; age-standardized prevalence 621.5 per 100,000 population). Of these patients, 24.0 million had active idiopathic epilepsy (prevalence 326.7 per 100,000 population). The prevalence of active epilepsy was found to increase with age, with peaks at ages 5–9 years (374.8) and >80 years (545.1). The global age-standardized mortality rate of idiopathic epilepsy was reported as 1.74 per 100,000 population, while age-standardized disability-adjusted life years (DALYs) was 182.6 per 100,000 population.

Between 1990 and 2016, there was a non-significant 6.0% decrease in the age-standardized prevalence of idiopathic epilepsy alongside a significant decrease in age-standardized mortality (24.5%) and DALY (19.4%) rates. One-third of the difference in age-standardized DALY rates between low and high SDI quintile countries was due to the greater severity of epilepsy in low-income settings, and the remaining two-thirds was due to a higher years of life lost (YLL) rate in low sociodemographic index (SDI) countries.

1.2.1.2 Comparison of the Prevalence, Morbidity, and Mortality of Epilepsy in Men and Women

Sex differences manifest across the entire continuum of brain development. From birth, males and females exhibit distinct brain volume variations, persisting across the lifespan, notably in seizure-prone areas like the hippocampus and amygdala.

Overall, males experience epilepsy marginally more frequently than females, a conclusion consistently supported by multiple epidemiological studies. The age-standardized prevalence of active idiopathic epilepsy is 329.3 per 100,000 population (280.3–381.2) in men and 318.9 per 100,000 population (271.1–369.4) in women and is similar among SDI quintiles. The global age-standardized mortality rate of idiopathic epilepsy is 1.40 per 100,000 population in women and 2.09 per 100,000 population in men. Age-standardized DALYs are 163.6 per 100,000 population for women and 201.2 per 100,000 population for men. The higher DALY rates in men are due to higher YLL rates compared with women.

Numerous factors, including lifestyle and environmental influences, may explain the observed sex differences in epilepsy. However, epilepsies are heterogeneous, exhibiting variations in symptoms, causes, and sex-specific prevalence.

Some studies have shown inconsistent rates of generalized tonic-clonic seizures across sexes; some studies indicate higher rates in males, while others report no significant difference or increased rates in females. These discrepancies could result from small study populations or diverse reporting practices internationally. The Epilepsy Phenome/Genome Project data suggests atonic seizures are more prevalent in males, contrasting with generalized genetic epilepsies like juvenile myoclonic epilepsy, which are more frequent in females. Certain X-linked conditions, such as Rett syndrome, predominantly affect females due to higher male mortality in utero or early life. Conversely, Fragile X syndrome-related seizures are reportedly more common in males. Reports on early life epilepsies like infantile spasms are varied, with some indicating a male predominance and others showing no significant sex disparity.

1.2.1.3 Characteristics of Epidemiological Data on Epilepsy in Women

Epilepsy is notably prevalent among women worldwide, with an incidence of 6.85 per 1000. Studies indicate that childhood and juvenile absence epilepsy are more common in females than males.

Managing epilepsy in women poses distinct challenges due to the impact of hormonal fluctuations on seizure control and the metabolism of antiseizure medications. For instance, catamenial epilepsy, which is characterized by seizure patterns linked to the menstrual cycle, affects approximately one-third of women with epilepsy. Research on catamenial epilepsy continues, yet a conclusive treatment is still out of reach. This is due to the ambiguous outcomes of existing studies. For instance, a placebo-controlled trial revealed that the percentage of women with catamenial epilepsy experiencing at least a 50% decrease in seizure frequency over 3 months of cyclic progesterone therapy did not differ significantly from the reduction seen in women without catamenial epilepsy during a similar baseline period.

1.2.2 Social Psychology of Women with Epilepsy

Although the prevalence of epilepsy and treatment approaches are similar for women and men, WWE have many social and physiological sex-specific problems. For example, women are more likely to experience seizure patterns related to hormonal cycles and are at risk of reproductive alterations and pregnancy complications.

1.2.2.1 Stigma

Stigma represents one of the most difficult challenges associated with epilepsy. In a study by Jane et al., all participants reported having experienced seizures that caused fall-related injuries such as fractures, burns, cuts, and bruises. They also reported that the seizures were occasionally associated with fecal and/or urinary incontinence as well as exposure of their body parts, which caused them much shame (von Gaudecker et al. 2017). Such stigma is felt particularly acutely by teenagers (MacLeod and Austin 2003; Zupanc and Haut 2008). Epilepsy are more often poor and marginalized members of society and have lower self-esteem, greater social isolation, poorer psychological health, lower quality of life, and worse epilepsy control that reducing stigma could improve quality of life for adolescents with epilepsy, and the World Health Organization's "Out of the Shadows" campaign in 1997 highlighted the above-mentioned issues efforts stigma is a very real, ongoing issue facing patients with epilepsy (Reynolds 2001).

Austin et al. surveyed epilepsy familiarity, knowledge, and perceptions about stigma in a large population of high school students; the majority of students believed that having epilepsy could "make you unpopular" and lead to being picked on or bullied in school (Austin et al. 2002) (Table 1.1). Only one-third of respondents would date someone with epilepsy. Although the majority of students stated that they would want a friend with epilepsy to tell them about their condition, fewer

Table 1.1 Percentages for stigma items in a study by Austin et al.

	Yes	Not sure	No	Do not know
If you had epilepsy, would you tell your friends?	46	31	10	14
Do you think having epilepsy would make you unpopular?	13	31	42	14
Do you think kids with epilepsy are likely to get picked on or bullied more than other kids?	37	26	24	13
If a friend had epilepsy, would you want him or her to tell you?	69	15	5	11

Questionnaire administered to a general population of high school students

would in turn reveal the same diagnosis to their friends. In fact, Westbrook et al. demonstrated that 70–85% of adolescents with epilepsy do not reveal their diagnosis to their friends, or rarely discuss it (Westbrook et al. 1992). Despite these realities, there are reassuring findings as well. In the study by Westbrook et al., most adolescents did not feel stigmatized or perceive that epilepsy affected their ability to have friendships or to date; however, many of the adolescents did not inform their friends about their epilepsy diagnosis, which may have contributed to this perceived lack of stigma. Furthermore, in developing the Quality of Life in Epilepsy Inventory for Adolescents-48 (QOLIE-AD-48), Cramer et al. reported an overall high quality of life (QoL) with low levels of stigma in their adolescent cohort. Interestingly, the presence and effect of stigma in adolescence has not generally been associated with gender (Cramer et al. 1999).

However, across the lifespan, the stigma of epilepsy and its consequences appear to be greater for women than for men. WWE experience more difficulties in attaining and maintaining marriages than do men, especially in low-income countries where socioeconomic and cultural constraints negatively influence recognition and acceptance of the disease. Married WWE face unique challenges and often encounter greater stigma compared to their male counterparts. This may stem from various factors, including blame for not disclosing their condition, discrimination from their spouse's family, fear of rejection by in-laws, negative perceptions from the spouse and relatives, adverse outcomes during pregnancy, and the threat of divorce. Consequently, stigma is identified as a major obstacle in managing epilepsy.

1.2.2.2 Mental Health

Patients with epilepsy exhibit a high rate of psychiatric comorbidities. Depression occurs in 11–80% of individuals with epilepsy, a stark contrast to the 4.9–17% prevalence in the broader population (Jones et al. 2010; Kerr et al. 2011). Anxiety is also more common among epilepsy patients, affecting 15–20%, compared to 5–7% in the general population. Psychiatric comorbidities are notably more common in epilepsy than in chronic diseases such as cancer, diabetes, or asthma. Moreover, individuals with psychiatric issues like depression are at increased risk for epilepsy, indicating a possible shared pathophysiological basis between psychiatric ailments and epilepsy.

The etiology of psychiatric problems in epilepsy is complex and includes genetic vulnerability, reaction to life events including the epilepsy itself, personality, age at disease onset of epilepsy, duration of epilepsy, temporal lobe epilepsy subtype, and the presence of family history of psychiatric illness (particularly depression). For example, patients with an age of disease onset less than 25 years have been shown to be more depressed than those aged over 25 years at disease onset; this relationship may result from the fact that people diagnosed with epilepsy at a younger age may not have sufficient life experience to cope with the stigma and discrimination associated with epilepsy, contributing to comorbid psychiatric illnesses (Mar Htwe et al. 2023). Depression is also associated with social stigma. A recent study suggested that patients who felt stigmatized by their epilepsy diagnosis were at increased risk of depression. Depression affects treatment compliance and this can lead to the development of a vicious cycle. Patients that, due to prejudices, are subjected to social or psychological isolation can stop seeking good health; self-management is negatively affected and coping with the disease becomes difficult. The perceived stigma level increases in patients who cannot manage their disease. From a different perspective, some personality studies indicate that introversion, pessimism, and avoidance are prevalent traits among individuals with epilepsy, who often suffer from increased anxiety and depression. The level of perceived stigma may be amplified in these individuals due to their negative outlook on the condition. Anxiety and depression are frequent psychiatric issues in those with epilepsy. Gender also plays a role in psychiatric comorbidities, with females experiencing anxiety and depression at twice the rate of males, a pattern that holds true for those with epilepsy. A retrospective study revealed depression rates of 15.5% in males and 26.8% in females with epilepsy, while anxiety disorders were present in 9.65% of males and 17.4% of females with the condition (Christian et al. 2020). As noted above, it is more difficult for WWE to attain and maintain a marriage. As a result, many WWE do not benefit from the protective effects of marriage and lack important emotional support from family members. A study by Beghi et al. confirmed the assumption that WWE of childbearing age are at high risk of depression (Beghi et al. 2004). Beghørk et al. also reported psychiatric disease in the peripartum period in WWE and identified peripartum depression, anxiety, and fear of birth as the most clinically relevant conditions (Bjørk et al. 2015a). Specifically, the point prevalence of depression from the second trimester of pregnancy to 6 months postpartum ranged from 16% to 35% in WWE (compared to 9–12% in controls), with the highest estimates recorded in pregnancy and in the perinatal period. Furthermore, anxiety symptoms 6 months postpartum were reported by 10% of WWE and 5% of controls. Fear of birth symptoms were increased in primiparous WWE compared with controls, and the main associated risk factors were previous psychiatric disease abuse, ASM polytherapy, high seizure frequency, and long duration of epilepsy were the main risk factors (Thome-Souza et al. 2004; Cavanna et al. 2010; Eddy et al. 2012; Meador et al. 2022).

1.2.2.3 Sexual Dysfunction

Men and WWE are more susceptible to reproductive endocrine disorders than the general population. Research on the pathophysiology of these comorbidities has concentrated on the hypothalamic-pituitary-gonadal (HPG) axis. This axis connects the brain to fertility and reproduction control across mammalian species. In the hypothalamus, gonadotropin-releasing hormone (GnRH) neurons release GnRH peptides, prompting the anterior pituitary's gonadotrope cells to produce luteinizing hormone (LH) and follicle-stimulating hormone (FSH). These hormones, acting on the gonads, promote gametogenesis and sex steroid hormone production in both genders. LH and FSH levels are detectable in the bloodstream, making them practical markers for HPG axis activity in humans, including epilepsy patients. Notably, LH and FSH are secreted in pulses, and variations in their pulsatility and basal levels are key indicators of hypothalamic-pituitary axis disruptions in individuals with epilepsy. Studies have noted changes in LH pulse frequency in patients with epilepsy, though findings are inconsistent. Additionally, a common observation is the diminished LH response to external GnRH administration, coupled with altered average LH or FSH levels. These fluctuations in gonadotropin levels hint at changes in brain activity affecting the pituitary's response to GnRH and the synthesis and release of gonadotropins, especially in those with temporal lobe epilepsy (TLE).

Sex steroid hormones, including estradiol, progesterone, and testosterone, significantly impact neural activity and seizure occurrence. Consequently, deviations from normal sex steroid production and secretion can greatly affect seizure management. Notably, individuals with epilepsy frequently exhibit altered levels of these hormones. While such changes are commonly side effects of ASMs, especially valproic acid, epilepsy, and seizures themselves have been linked to hormonal fluctuations, particularly in testosterone levels.

Another pituitary hormone critical to correct regulation of HPG axis function is prolactin (PRL), which is synthesized under dopaminergic control from the hypothalamic arcuate nucleus to the posterior pituitary. This connection facilitates a direct link between brain seizure activity and PRL secretion. Elevated PRL can inhibit the GnRH-LH axis, suggesting hyperprolactinemia as a potential cause of reproductive dysfunction in epilepsy patients. Studies on PRL levels in WWE show mixed results, with some indicating increases and others showing no change. In men with TLE, about 10% exhibit hyperprolactinemia, though some research notes immediate post-seizure PRL spikes without average level alterations. Postictal PRL elevation has been observed regardless of sex, particularly in TLE patients. Consequently, measuring serum PRL levels shortly after seizures is proposed as a diagnostic method to differentiate epileptic seizures from psychogenic non-epileptic seizures.

One of the most notable gender disparities in epilepsy is the cyclical pattern of seizure exacerbations that WWE often experience during specific menstrual cycle phases. Both focal epilepsies, like TLE, and some primary generalized epilepsies, such as juvenile myoclonic epilepsy, may show catamenial exacerbations. Catamenial epilepsy affects 25–70% of women of reproductive age with epilepsy; this variance is due to differing definitions and diagnostic criteria. Hormonal cycles cause neurosteroid level changes, leading to seizure increases in catamenial epilepsy during certain menstrual phases. This condition occurs in both ovulatory and anovulatory cycles. One study found that about 16.5% of participants had anovulatory cycles with an inadequate luteal phase. Three catamenial seizure types are identified: perimenstrual, periovulatory, and inadequate luteal phase, classified by the timing of seizure spikes relative to the menstrual cycle. Diagnosis involves charting menstruation and seizures, plus mid-luteal phase serum progesterone measurements to differentiate between normal and inadequate luteal phase cycles. The menstrual cycle is divided into four phases for diagnostic purposes: menstrual (days 24 to +3), follicular (days +4 to +9), ovulatory (days +10 to +16), and luteal (days +17 to 23). Recording seizures for at least two cycles, a twofold increase in seizures during a specific phase may diagnose catamenial epilepsy. The most common type, perimenstrual catamenial epilepsy, sees increased seizures from days 23 to 3. Despite conventional ASMs, many women continue to have cycle-related seizures, suggesting pharmacoresistance.

WWE often face additional health challenges, including anovulatory menstrual cycles, oligomenorrhea, polycystic ovaries, and polycystic ovarian syndrome (PCOS). Specifically, 10–25% of women with TLE are diagnosed with PCOS, which is significantly higher than the 4–6% prevalence in the general population. Additionally, 12% of women with TLE experience hypothalamic amenorrhea, surpassing the 1.5% rate among the general population. While these comorbidities have been extensively studied in TLE and other focal epilepsies, they are also prevalent in generalized epilepsy disorders. Although ASM treatment is known to contribute to reproductive endocrine issues, seizure activity itself is increasingly recognized as a primary factor. Notably, research has shown that women with left-sided TLE have higher PCOS rates, while those with right-sided TLE are more prone to hypothalamic amenorrhea and hypogonadotropic hypogonadism, including reduced sexual interest. These patterns suggest that specific brain regions affected by seizures may influence distinct reproductive endocrine disorders, highlighting the role of certain neural pathways in these altered functions.

WWE exhibit sexual dysfunction and diminished sexual arousal. Studies have found that many WWE have normal sexuality, but there is a significant fraction who have markedly decreased sexual desire and orgasmic dysfunction, including anorgasmia.

Some of the postulated mechanisms for sexual dysfunction and reduced fertility are related to the effect of epilepsy on reproductive hormones. GnRH cells in the preoptic area of the hypothalamus are vulnerable to seizure-induced injury. Dysfunction of GnRH cells is followed by the abnormal release of FSH and LH; this phenomenon is known as hypogonadotropic hypogonadism. In addition, ASMs may contribute to sexual dysfunction. Enzyme-inducing ASMs can lower libido by decreasing serum total testosterone, free androgen index, dehydroepiandrosterone sulfate, and estradiol levels, while increasing sex hormone-binding globulin. Withdrawal from carbamazepine, a commonly used ASM, has been shown to significantly increase total testosterone and free androgen index in both genders. Conversely, discontinuing valproate has minimal impact on these hormones. These findings suggest that ASM selection can influence sexual health-related hormones, with potential reversibility of effects. Valproate, known to suppress hepatic cytochrome P450 enzymes, negatively impacts sexual and thyroid functions and is linked to various conditions including hyperandrogenism, insulin resistance, weight gain, PCOS, menstrual irregularities, ovulatory failure, and infertility. Therefore, it is advisable to avoid valproate in women who may conceive. Non-enzyme-inducing ASMs like lamotrigine are preferable, as they have been associated with enhanced sexual functioning. Nonetheless, effective seizure management with ASMs can lead to improved sexual function, likely due to an overall better quality of life.

Recent research incorporating multiple logistic regression analyses reported that determinants of sexual dysfunction comprised the location of epilepsy foci, higher seizure frequency, and increased severity of depression and anxiety, but not lower androgen levels, epilepsy type, or ASM use (Hamed et al. 2020). Women with left-sided TLE exhibit elevated testosterone levels relative to those with right-sided TLE. Conversely, women with right-sided TLE show notably lower estradiol levels than their left-sided counterparts. These hormonal variations may indicate disruptions in specific neural pathways. The epilepsy literature suggests that seizures of right temporal origin are particularly associated with reproductive dysfunction and possibly even sexual ictal phenomenon; right temporal epileptic discharges in WWE are associated with hypogonadotropic hypogonadism that results in decreased sexual interest. A carefully conducted questionnaire study of sexual functioning in men and women with either right or left TLE found that sexual interest was decreased in patients with right TLE compared to left TLE in both genders, although most aspects of sexual performance were similar (Daniele et al. 1997). Ictal sexual behaviors and ictal orgasm have been specifically associated with right TLE. These findings suggest that right temporal resection could improve sexual functioning. Experimental evidence indicates that the right hypothalamus is predominant in the control of reproductive functioning. Therefore, a body of evidence from divergent sources, both clinical- and laboratory-based, suggest that right-sided epilepsy, and right TLE specifically, may be associated with a risk of sexual and reproductive dysfunction.

1.2.2.4 Quality of Life

People with epilepsy are predisposed to have lower QoL compared with healthy individuals (Fawale et al. 2014). Female gender is one of the most vital factors and highest risks for lower QoL in individuals with epilepsy. A recent Portuguese study reported that female gender is the second most significant contributor to the lower QoL in epilepsy (Silva et al. 2019). Clinical determinants including seizure type, seizure control, and type of ASMs received were significant contributors to the lower QoL in WWE. Seizure type was the most important clinical dimension influencing QoL in the study participants; individuals with generalized onset seizures report lower QoL than those with focal and unknown onset seizures. Srikanth et al. confirmed that education status also significantly affects QoL in epilepsy (Srikanth et al. 2021); illiterate individuals had lower QoL scores compared with literate individuals. Socioeconomic status (SES) also contributes to QoL. In a recent study, WWE of lower SES had lower QoL when compared with those of middle and high

SES. A study from south India reported that lower per capita income was associated with low QoL among people with epilepsy (Rakesh et al. 2012). The three pillars of health care quality (availability, accessibility, and affordability) vary in urban and rural communities. Furthermore, in rural areas, in addition to the three above-mentioned factors additional adversities exist, including stigma at multiple levels, which pose a profound challenge to individuals and adversely affect their QoL.

In addition, WWE face specific difficulties like sexual and reproductive dysfunction, pregnancy, lactation, menopause, contraception, and mental health aspects, in addition to many psychosocial issues such as a need to balance family life, conception, adverse pregnancy, poor drug adherence, and poor marital outcomes.

Three instruments are widely used to assess QoL in people with epilepsy: (1) the Quality of Life in Childhood Epilepsy (QOLCE) for individuals aged <11 years, (2) the QOLIE-AD-48 for individuals aged 11 to <18 years, and (3) the Quality of Life in Epilepsy Inventory-31-Problems (QOLIE-31-P) for individuals aged ≥18 years.

QOLCE is a parent-proxy report measure, meaning that it is completed by parents or caregivers on behalf of the child. The QOLCE was developed from an original questionnaire containing 91 items. Item analysis and validation led to a final questionnaire containing 76 items with 16 subscales covering five life function domains: physical function, social function, cognition, and emotional as well as behavioral well-being. The questionnaire was designed to capture the impact of epilepsy on different aspects of a child's life and provide valuable insights into their well-being. The QOLCE subscales correlate strongly with similar subscales in an existing generic health outcome measure, the Child Health Questionnaire (CHQ), and 12 of 16 subscales of the QOLCE correlate with a measure of seizure severity.

The QOLIE-AD-48 is a self-report measure specifically designed to assess the quality of life in adolescents (ages 11–18) with epilepsy. It contains 48 items in eight subscales: epilepsy impact (12 items), memory/concentration (10), attitudes toward epilepsy (4), physical functioning (5), stigma (6), social support (4), school behavior (4), and health perceptions (3). Each item in the QOLIE-AD-48 questionnaire is scored on a Likert scale, where adolescents rate their experiences and feelings in relation to each domain. The scores are then calculated to provide an overall assessment of the adolescent's QoL in relation to their epilepsy, with higher scores indicating better health-related QoL. The questionnaire can be completed in 15–20 min and provides information about a variety of issues pertinent to this age group.

The QOLIE-31-P is a self-report measure used to assess the impact of epilepsy on the QoL of individuals with epilepsy. It is designed for use in both adults and adolescents (ages 18 and older) with epilepsy. The QOLIE-31-P questionnaire comprises seven subscales covering general and epilepsy-specific domains, including 31 items that cover various domains related to the impact of epilepsy on an individual's life. These domains include seizure worry, overall QoL, emotional well-being, energy/fatigue, cognitive functioning, medication side effects, social functioning, and driving. Subscale and total scores can be calculated. The subscales are grouped into two factors: emotional/psychological effects (seizure worry, overall QOL, emotional well-being, energy/fatigue subscales) and medical/social effects (medication effects, work-driving-social limits, cognitive function subscales).

1.2.2.5 Quality of Life Characteristics in Adolescents, Women of Childbearing Age, and Menopausal Women with Epilepsy

1.2.2.5.1 Quality of Life in Adolescents

Adolescence is a period of growing independence accompanied by great physical and emotional changes. As their peers begin to explore the myriad developmental opportunities of the teenage years, adolescents with epilepsy wonder whether their condition will prevent them from driving, working, marrying, and having children. These concerns, superimposed on the medical burden of epilepsy, tend to significantly impact their health-related QoL. As mentioned above, adolescents with epilepsy are too young to deal with the stigma and discrimination associated with epilepsy, which ultimately leads to low QoL. Devinsky et al. reported that significant predictors of worse QoL included older age (14–17 years), more severe epilepsy, lower SES, and medication toxicity. Interestingly, younger adolescents (11–13 years) reported worse scores in the social support subscale, implying that social support networks may actually improve as adolescence progresses (Devinsky et al. 1999). Community-dwelling adolescents with epilepsy who are not followed in specialty clinics appear to have better overall QoL scores, reflective of better seizure control.

Gender effects are mixed. Female adolescents tend to describe a larger impact of epilepsy on their lives than males, and they appear to have worse QoL than males overall, describing more self-anxiety, worse self-image, and a higher epilepsy impact. However, there is evidence to suggest that females may fare better in peer relations and have less illness denial. While teenage females in general appear to have higher emotional distress related to chronic disorders, most are not given sufficient attention and they do not seek psychiatric help in larger numbers than their male counterparts.

1.2.2.5.2 Quality of Life in Women of Childbearing Age

Psychosocial problems are one of the important factors leading to impaired QoL in WWE, especially before and after pregnancy. This specific subpopulation is particularly likely to develop depression in relation to the complications of pregnancy, which tend to be higher than expected in the general population as a consequence of epilepsy and ASMs, with subsequent impairment of health-related QOL (Beghi et al. 2004). In the MoBa study, 706 WWE completed anxiety and depression questionnaires during pregnancy and up to 36 months postpartum (Bjørk et al. 2015b). When compared to 106,511 women without epilepsy and 8372 with other chronic conditions, those with epilepsy reported higher instances of depression or anxiety but were less frequently prescribed antidepressants. Factors such as a history of anxiety, depression, and ASM treatment increased the risk. Recovery from anxiety and depression was adversely impacted by prior physical and sexual abuse, as well as anxiety and depression. Additionally, epilepsy correlated with a higher occurrence of binge-eating disorder and negative body image during pregnancy. Quality of life data from the MoBa study, which included 719 WWE and 101,546 without, revealed that epilepsy was linked to lower overall life satisfaction, self-esteem, and challenging socioeconomic conditions, including single parenthood, financial struggles, limited education, and unemployment both during and after pregnancy.

Santos et al. reported that women of childbearing age with epilepsy tend to have lower QoL than those without epilepsy, suggesting that the clinical variables associated with worsening of health-related QoL were seizure control and the adverse effects of ASMs (Srikanth et al. 2021; Santos et al. 2018).

During pregnancy, most WWE, including those with catamenial epilepsy, see an improvement in seizures or remain seizure-free. For instance, in the European and International Registry of Antiseizure Medications and Pregnancy, 66% (2521 out of 3806) pregnancies in WWE were seizure-free. Specifically, 73.6% (1096 out of 1491) of pregnancies in women with genetic generalized epilepsies had no seizures. However, a smaller proportion, 59.5% (1063 out of 1786), of women with localization-related epilepsies experienced seizure freedom. Seizure control worsened in 15.8% (589 out of 3735) of women during the second and third trimesters compared to the first. A U.S. study indicated higher mortality rates during pregnancy for WWE (80 deaths per 100,000 pregnancies) versus those without (6 deaths per 100,000 pregnancies). In the UK, epilepsy is a leading indirect cause of maternal death, often due to sudden unexpected death in epilepsy. Therefore, it's crucial to enhance seizure control and offer counseling and support to pregnant women with uncontrolled seizures (Stephen et al. 2019).

Pregnancy induces physiological changes that can alter the absorption, distribution, metabolism, and elimination of ASMs. The levels of lamotrigine, levetiracetam, topiramate, zonisamide, and oxcarbazepine in the blood may decrease as pregnancy advances. The sex of the fetus and genetic variations in uridine 5′-diphospho-glucuronosyltransferase (UGT)—the enzyme primarily responsible for metabolizing lamotrigine—can influence lamotrigine levels. A study of 47 pregnancies in 40 WWE showed that those with female fetuses had more significant reductions in lamotrigine concentration-to-dose (C:D) ratios than those with male fetuses. Women with the *UGT1A4 142TG (3) polymorphism experienced a less marked decrease in lamotrigine C:D ratios in the third trimester compared to those without the polymorphism. Similarly, individuals homozygous for UGT2B7 802TT had significantly lower C:D ratios in the first and third trimesters than heterozygous carriers. Therapeutic drug monitoring is beneficial for adjusting ASM dosages during pregnancy. While conclusive evidence is lacking, UK guidelines suggest maintaining ASM therapy throughout pregnancy and breastfeeding to ensure seizure control and prevent tonic-clonic seizures. Valproate carries the highest risk of congenital malformations, with the danger increasing as the daily dose rises from 500 to 750 mg. Genetic predispositions, like a family history of neural tube defects or individual susceptibility, may also contribute to the risk of congenital malformations. Valproate use during pregnancy is linked to poorer neurodevelopmental outcomes in children, with increased developmental delays in cognition, motor skills, and language compared to children of untreated WWE. Children whose mothers took valproate had a lower average intelligence quotient (IQ) score of 97, versus 105 for carbamazepine, 108 for lamotrigine, and 108 for phenytoin. Higher doses of valproate (>800 mg/day) resulted in an adjusted mean IQ that was 9.7 points lower, with significant deficits in verbal, non-verbal, and spatial abilities, and an eightfold increase in the need for educational support. These children also scored lower in Welsh national tests for math and science between ages 7 and 16, but not in languages. In utero exposure to valproate also raised the risk of autism spectrum disorder, dyspraxia, and ADHD. Therefore, valproate is best avoided in women who may become pregnant.

Research indicates that WWE face a heightened risk of pregnancy complications. Data from pregnancy registries reveal that spontaneous abortions occur more frequently in women exposed to ASMs, including those with epilepsy, compared to those not on ASMs or without epilepsy. Additionally, these women are more likely to undergo pregnancy termination. The incidence of preeclampsia is also elevated in WWE. Obesity is more prevalent among pregnant WWE, increasing the likelihood of cesarean delivery and excessive bleeding, especially when compared to overweight women without epilepsy and those with epilepsy who have a normal body mass index. Due to these risks, it is recommended that WWE receive specialist-led obstetric care and hospital admission in case of complications.

In addition, Srikanth et al. reported that significant sociodemographic determinants of lower QoL include illiteracy, being married, unemployed, and having children.

1.2.2.5.3 Quality of Life in Menopausal Women

Limited research exists on the relationship between epilepsy and menopause. Findings from two surveys indicate that WWE may enter perimenopause and menopause prematurely. One study linked a higher total number of seizures with an onset of menopause 3–4 years earlier than usual, particularly in women who had over 20 seizures (Vélez-Ruiz and Pennell 2016; Harden et al. 2016). Additionally, WWE who experience seizures have been found to have lower levels of anti-Müllerian hormone, which reflects ovarian reserve, compared to those without seizures. It is important for WWE to understand the potential consequences of early menopause, such as a reduced fertility period. Upon reaching menopause, considerations around stopping contraception and addressing bone health become pertinent.

During perimenopause, the frequency of seizures may rise due to swift fluctuations in estrogen and progesterone levels. Post-menopause, seizure occurrences might diminish, potentially because of increased estrone levels, which have demonstrated seizure-reducing effects in catamenial epilepsy patients and in research models. A survey of 16 women with catamenial epilepsy history revealed that 69% (11 women) experienced fewer seizures. This indicates that internal sex steroid hormone changes may affect brain excitability. Present treatment approaches emphasize fine-tuning ASM protocols. As insights into the hormone-seizure connection during menopause deepen, potential improvements in epilepsy therapies for this life stage could emerge.

Exogenous hormones may affect seizure patterns in menopausal WWE. In a randomized, placebo-controlled study involving 15 women on hormone replacement therapy (HRT) with conjugated equine estrogens and medroxyprogesterone acetate, 40% experienced an increase in seizure frequency and severity, suggesting a dose-related response. Consequently, HRT is generally discouraged. Additionally, estrogen-containing HRT can lower lamotrigine levels, implying that monitoring lamotrigine concentrations might be beneficial. Dosage adjustments may be necessary to maintain seizure control.

During menopause, bone turnover rates increase, accelerating bone loss and decreasing bone mineral density. This can lead to fractures, causing chronic pain, disability, reduced quality of life, and even death. ASMs, especially those that enzyme-inducing enzymes, are linked to lower bone mineral density, making post-menopausal WWE more prone to fractures. The exact causes are complex and likely multifactorial, with poor mobility and intellectual disability also contributing to the risk. Bone loss may begin before menopause in women taking ASMs. A UK study noted that among 10,000 WWE (median age 48.2 years) who used enzyme-inducing ASMs for a year, there were 48 additional fractures. Other ASMs like valproate are also associated with lower bone mineral density. In a group of 50 adults with epilepsy on valproate, bone mineral density was significantly lower compared to those without epilepsy. Managing low bone mineral density in WWE is challenging. Some may need enzyme-inducing ASMs to control seizures, and switching to another medication with a potentially lower risk of bone density reduction could lead to seizure-related fractures.

1.2.2.6 Principles and Components of Social and Psychological Care for Female Patients with Epilepsy

WWE encounter various challenges throughout their lives. Younger women often need guidance on managing seizures in relation to their menstrual cycle, as well as advice on contraception, fertility, and pregnancy.

Older women may seek information on seizures during menopause and the impact of ASMs on bone mineral density. The exact causes of catamenial epilepsy are not fully understood, and current research indicates that progesterone supplements may not be suitable for most affected women. There is a reported lack of knowledge among WWE regarding critical pregnancy and childbirth concerns, and their use of hormonal contraception is lower than that of the general female population, highlighting a need for better contraceptive and preconception counseling. Although most WWE experience positive pregnancy outcomes, studies indicate increased morbidity and mortality rates compared to pregnant women without epilepsy. Physiological changes during pregnancy necessitate adjustments in ASM dosages, particularly for lamotrigine, levetiracetam, topiramate, zonisamide, and oxcarbazepine. Maternal folic acid supplementation has shown neurodevelopmental benefits for the offspring of WWE, yet further research is needed to determine its role in preventing congenital malformations and to establish optimal dosing. WWE also have a higher likelihood of psychiatric comorbidities during the peripartum period. Therefore, comprehensive postnatal counseling is essential to address breastfeeding, seizure management, and ASM considerations.

WWE experience early perimenopause and menopause more frequently than those without the condition, yet the exact causes are unclear. Antiseizure medications contribute to bone density reduction, increasing the risk of bone loss. Epilepsy can negatively impact social skills, relationships, and employment opportunities, but the specific mechanisms and potential interventions require further research. Understanding the processes that cause catamenial epilepsy is crucial for developing targeted treatments. The creation of effective, nonhormonal contraceptives or those without drug interactions would provide better options for WWE, potentially leading to more contraceptive use and fewer unintended pregnancies. Investigating the genetic and mechanistic origins of congenital malformations and neurodevelopmental issues associated with antiseizure medications will enhance preconception counseling for WWE.

1.3 Overview of Global Cohort Studies of Women with Epilepsy

Ding Ding

1.3.1 Clinical Cohort Studies: Designs and Methodologies

There is a lack of high-level clinical evidence to support drug treatments for female patients with epilepsy during pregnancy, and it is difficult to include a large enough sample in a single-center study; furthermore, it is not in line with medical ethics to conduct randomized controlled trials on patients with epilepsy during pregnancy. Therefore, a multi-country, multi-center cooperative epileptic pregnancy registry system has emerged. Table 1.2 demonstrated the major cohorts of pregnant women with epilepsy worldwide. At present, the three largest international epileptic pregnancy registries are the UK and Ireland Epilepsy and Pregnancy Registers (UKIEPR), the North American AED Pregnancy Registry, and the International Registry of Antiseizure medications and Pregnancy (EURAP). And China, Australia, and India registries are contributing to EURAP.

The UKIEPR combines the UK Epilepsy and Pregnancy Register (UKEPR), established in 1996, and the Irish Epilepsy and Pregnancy Register, established in 2001, which were merged in 2007; more than 8000 cases of epilepsy in pregnancy were enrolled by 2014. Covering roughly one-third of all epileptic pregnancies in the UK and Ireland, it is one of the earliest and largest independent epilepsy and pregnancy registries. The UKIEPR aims to study the safety of all anti-epileptic drugs during pregnancy, and relies on pregnancy registration by health care workers or epilepsy patients themselves, providing the prospective inclusion of all pregnant epilepsy patients, regardless of whether the patient takes ASMs. Information

Table 1.2 Description of major cohorts of pregnant women with epilepsy worldwide

Registries	Setting	Study design	Methods of enrollment	Inclusion criteria	Outcome assessment	ASM drug levels
EURAP (Tomson et al. 2018)	International	Prospective/ retrospective	Through networks of reporting physicians	Pregnancies with ASM exposure at time of conception	Central classification by blinded teratologists based on reports from physicians	Not recorded
North America (Pennell et al. 2022)	U.S. and Canada	Prospective/ retrospective	Patient self-enrollment	Women taking ASMs for any reason during pregnancy	Review of medical records by blinded teratologist, direct communication with mother/physician when needed	Recorded
United Kingdom and Ireland (Campbell et al. 2014)	United Kingdom and Ireland	Prospective	Through physicians, nurses, and patient self-enrollment	Women with epilepsy with/without ASMs first trimester	Abnormal outcomes classified by one clinical geneticist based on medical records	Not recorded
Australia (contributes to EURAP) (Vajda et al. 2022)	Australia	Prospective/ retrospective	Patient self-enrollment	Women with epilepsy with/without ASMs first trimester	Based on review of medical records	Not recorded
Kerala (contributes to EURAP) (Seshachala et al. 2021)	India	Prospective	Referred by physicians, gynecologist and patients self-referral	Women with active epilepsy with/without AEDs. Women on AEDs in first trimester for other indication	Direct evaluation by reporting physician supplemented by echocardiography and ultrasonography	Not recorded
China (contributes to EURAP) (Li et al. 2023)	China	Prospective/ retrospective	Through networks of reporting physicians	Women with epilepsy with/without ASMs first trimester	Based on review of medical records	Recorded

collected includes demographic data, cause of epilepsy, type and frequency of seizures, ASMs taken from 3 months before pregnancy to pregnancy, use of other medications such as folic acid during pregnancy, pregnancy history, relevant family history, prenatal exam results, and pregnancy outcomes. Follow-up data are provided by the patient's family physician from the time of registration until 3 months after delivery.

The North American AED Pregnancy Registry, established in 1997 at Massachusetts General Hospital in Boston, USA, includes all women taking ASMs during pregnancy in the United States and Canada. The purpose of this registry is to study the incidence of major abnormalities in the offspring of women who take one or more ASMs for any reason, with a particular focus on the pregnancy safety of new ASMs. This is the first epilepsy registry to be established by a hospital, and 10,200 pregnancies have been registered as of May 2016. Collected information includes the start and end time of ASMs, dose, frequency of administration, and medication adjustment for each type, as well as demographic information about the pregnant person, smoking history, alcohol history, drug abuse history, other drug use history, family history, and prenatal exam results. For patients with epilepsy, data on the number and type of seizures during pregnancy are collected. Telephone follow-up commences at 7 months of gestation and again at 8–12 weeks postpartum, and information is extracted from the patient's medical records in about 60% of cases.

The EURAP was established in 1999 by a consortium of several European epilepsy research groups. Subsequently, thanks to the support of the International League Against Epilepsy (ILAE), it has rapidly developed into a worldwide epilepsy registry, with more than 1500 collaborators from 42 countries joining EURAP and completing more than 23,200 pregnancy registrations. Pregnancy registration information is collected by clinicians through a web-based registration system and aggregated to a central database located in Milan, Italy. The EURAP includes all patients who have taken ASMs during pregnancy and aims to explore and compare the safety of new ASMs pregnancies. The EURAP also aims to assess the long-term effects of intrauterine ASM exposure on maternal cognitive function. Follow-up is conducted during the first, second, and third trimesters as well as 12 months after delivery. Data collected include information on demographics, type of epilepsy, frequency of seizures, comorbidities, major congenital malformations, family history, type of antiseizure medication therapy used, dosage, and other risk factors.

Numerous guidelines for the management of women with epilepsy have been developed from studies based on large international epileptic pregnancy registries, and the Task Force on Women and Pregnancy of the International League Against Epilepsy conducted a survey on the use of guidelines or recommendations for the management of women with epilepsy during pregnancy. The results showed that at least 20% of the guidelines did not include information on possible risks to cognitive development, information on the specific risks of specific anti-epileptic drugs, and no advice on the choice of anti-epileptic drugs. Furthermore, 91% reported that folic acid supplementation was recommended, but recommended dosages ranged from 0.4 to 4 mg/day or more; 34% of the reports did not include recommendations for monitoring drug levels during pregnancy, and 19% did not include breastfeeding guidelines. As a result, up-to-date and globally applicable recommendations for the management of pregnancy epilepsy are still lacking.

Although large-scale international studies on epileptic pregnancy registries have provided medical evidence for the management of female patients to a large extent, through summarizing the characteristics of the above-mentioned large-scale international pregnancy registries we identified some limitations in the current global cohort studies of women with epilepsy. First, the current global cohort studies of women with epilepsy mainly focus on the safety of drugs during pregnancy, including the correlation between the type and dose of drugs during pregnancy and offspring malformations as well as other adverse outcomes in the offspring. However, there are few studies on the relationship between the ASMs and adverse offspring outcomes relating to breast milk, and on the relationship between the ASMs and adverse pregnancy events (such as spontaneous abortion, prenatal bleeding, gestational hypertension, and preterm birth). In addition, current research on the outcome of pregnancy in women with epilepsy mainly focuses on the mother and the living offspring, and the relative lack of research on the monitoring of fetal growth and development during pregnancy in female patients with epilepsy has led to the partial neglect of those who choose to terminate pregnancy early for various reasons. Currently, according to the results of the global cohort studies of women with epilepsy, the management goals of epilepsy control before pregnancy (that is, at least how long is required to achieve seizure control before pregnancy) are currently not unified. The timing and dosage of folic acid to be administered in these patients remains controversial. In terms of data sources, the current large pregnancy registries mainly cover Western countries such as Europe, America, and Australia, and data from Asian countries are lacking. Therefore, there is still a large gap in the global cohort studies of women with epilepsy. Finally, with changes in the types of antiseizure medications available, new drugs have increasingly replaced the older generation of antiseizure medications, and the use of new antiseizure medications in pregnant women has gradually increased. Current studies have found that as the use of newer ASMs has increased and the use of older ASMs decreased, the prevalence of congenital malformations in the offspring of WWE has decreased by 27%. However, because pregnancy registries studying the teratogenic risks of new antiseizure medications remain small, it is not yet possible to determine the effects of the new antiseizure medications themselves on pregnancy.

References

Austin JK, Shafer PO, Deering JB. Epilepsy familiarity, knowledge, and perceptions of stigma: report from a survey of adolescents in the general population. Epilepsy Behav. 2002;3(4):368–75. https://doi.org/10.1016/s1525-5050(02)00042-2.

Beghi E, Roncolato M, Visonà G. Depression and altered quality of life in women with epilepsy of childbearing age. Epilepsia. 2004;45(1):64–70. https://doi.org/10.1111/j.0013-9580.2004.56502.x.

Bjørk MH, Veiby G, Engelsen BA, et al. Depression and anxiety during pregnancy and the postpartum period in women with epilepsy: a review of frequency, risks and recommendations for treatment. Seizure. 2015a;28:39–45. https://doi.org/10.1016/j.seizure.2015.02.016.

Bjørk MH, Veiby G, Reiter SC, et al. Depression and anxiety in women with epilepsy during pregnancy and after delivery: a prospective population-based cohort study on frequency, risk factors, medication, and prognosis. Epilepsia. 2015b;56(1):28–39. https://doi.org/10.1111/epi.12884.

Campbell E, Kennedy F, Russell A, Smithson WH, Parsons L, Morrison PJ, Liggan B, Irwin B, Delanty N, Hunt SJ, Craig J, Morrow J. Malformation risks of antiepileptic drug monotherapies in pregnancy: updated results from the UK and Ireland Epilepsy and Pregnancy Registers. J Neurol Neurosurg Psychiatry. 2014;85(9):1029–34. https://doi.org/10.1136/jnnp-2013-306318.

Cavanna AE, Ali F, Rickards HE, et al. Behavioral and cognitive effects of anti-epileptic drugs. Discov Med. 2010;9(45):138–44.

Christian CA, Reddy DS, Maguire J, et al. Sex differences in the epilepsies and associated comorbidities: implications for use and development of pharmacotherapies. Pharmacol Rev. 2020;72(4):767–800. https://doi.org/10.1124/pr.119.017392.

Cramer JA, Westbrook LE, Devinsky O, et al. Development of the quality of life in epilepsy inventory for adolescents: the QOLIE-AD-48. Epilepsia. 1999;40(8):1114–21. https://doi.org/10.1111/j.1528-1157.1999.tb00828.x.

Daniele A, Azzoni A, Bizzi A, et al. Sexual behavior and hemispheric laterality of the focus in patients with temporal lobe epilepsy. Biol Psychiatry. 1997;42(7):617–24. https://pubmed.ncbi.nlm.nih.gov/9376458/.

Devinsky O, Westbrook L, Cramer J, et al. Risk factors for poor health-related quality of life in adolescents with epilepsy. Epilepsia. 1999;40(12):1715–20. https://doi.org/10.1111/j.1528-1157.1999.tb01588.x.

Eddy CM, Rickards HE, Cavanna AE. Behavioral adverse effects of antiepileptic drugs in epilepsy. J Clin Psychopharmacol. 2012;32(3):362–75. https://doi.org/10.1097/JCP.0b013e318253a186.

Fawale MB, Owolabi MO, Ogunniyi A. Effects of seizure severity and seizure freedom on the health-related quality of life of an African population of people with epilepsy. Epilepsy Behav. 2014;32:9–14. https://doi.org/10.1016/j.yebeh.2013.12.026.

GBD 2016 Epilepsy Collaborators. Global, regional, and national burden of epilepsy, 1990-2016: a systematic analysis for the Global Burden of Disease Study 2016. Lancet Neurol. 2019;18(4):357–75. https://doi.org/10.1016/S1474-4422(18)30454-X.

Hamed SA, Attiah FA, Gabra RH, et al. Sexual functions in women with focal epilepsy: relationship to demographic, clinical, hormonal and psychological variables. Clin Neurol Neurosurg. 2020;191:105697. https://doi.org/10.1016/j.clineuro.2020.105697.

Harden CL, Pennell PB, French JA, et al. Anti-mullerian hormone is higher in seizure-free women with epilepsy compared to those with ongoing seizures. Epilepsy Res. 2016;127:66–71. https://doi.org/10.1016/j.eplepsyres.2016.08.003.

Jones R, Rickards H, Cavanna AE. The prevalence of psychiatric disorders in epilepsy: a critical review of the evidence. Funct Neurol. 2010;25(4):191–4.

Kerr MP, Mensah S, Besag F, et al. International consensus clinical practice statements for the treatment of neuropsychiatric conditions associated with epilepsy. Epilepsia. 2011;52(11):2133–8. https://doi.org/10.1111/j.1528-1167.2011.03276.x.

Li R, Chen Q, Cao X, Yan H, Wang P, Huang Q, Li X, Chen F, Li Y, Kong Q, Guo C, Zhang Q, Hong Q, Liu Y, Xiong X, Han Y, Xiao X, Wang K, Wu X, Zhu X, Zhang Q, Chen L. Pregnancy characteristics and adverse outcomes in offspring of women with epilepsy: a prospective registry study from Mainland China. Front Neurol. 2023;14:1195003. https://doi.org/10.3389/fneur.2023.1195003.

MacLeod JS, Austin JK. Stigma in the lives of adolescents with epilepsy: a review of the literature. Epilepsy Behav. 2003;4(2):112–7. https://doi.org/10.1016/s1525-5050(03)00007-6.

Mar Htwe Z, Lae Phyu W, Zar Nyein Z, et al. Correlation between depression and perceived stigma among people living with epilepsy. Epilepsy Behav. 2023;146:109372. https://doi.org/10.1016/j.yebeh.2023.109372.

Meador KJ, Stowe ZN, Brown C, et al. Prospective cohort study of depression during pregnancy and the postpartum period in women with epilepsy vs control groups. Neurology. 2022;99(15):e1573–83. https://doi.org/10.1212/WNL.0000000000200958.

Pennell PB, Karanam A, Meador KJ, Gerard E, Kalayjian L, Penovich P, Matthews A, McElrath TM, Birnbaum AK, MONEAD Study Group. Antiseizure medication concentrations during pregnancy: results from the maternal outcomes and neurodevelopmental effects of antiepileptic drugs (MONEAD) study. JAMA Neurol. 2022;79(4):370–9. https://doi.org/10.1001/jamaneurol.2021.5487.

Rakesh PS, Ramesh R, Rachel P, et al. Quality of life among people with epilepsy: a cross-sectional study from rural southern India. Natl Med J India. 2012;25(5):261–4.

Reynolds EH. ILAE/IBE/WHO global campaign "out of the shadows": global and regional developments. Epilepsia. 2001;42(8):1094–100. https://doi.org/10.1046/j.1528-1157.2001.0420081094.x.

Santos AMC, Castro-Lima H, Matos MAA, et al. Quality of life among women with epilepsy during their reproductive years. Epilepsy Behav. 2018;85:10–3. https://doi.org/10.1016/j.yebeh.2018.04.028.

Seshachala BB, Jose M, Lathikakumari AM, Murali S, Kumar AS, Thomas SV. Valproate usage in pregnancy: an audit from the Kerala Registry of Epilepsy and Pregnancy. Epilepsia. 2021;62(5):1141–7. https://doi.org/10.1111/epi.16882.

Silva B, Canas-Simião H, Cordeiro S, et al. Determinants of quality of life in patients with drug-resistant focal epilepsy. Epilepsy Behav. 2019;100:106525. https://doi.org/10.1016/j.yebeh.2019.106525.

Srikanth P, Vranda MN, Thomas PT, et al. Quality of life and stigma among women with epilepsy during their reproductive years. J Epilepsy Res. 2021;11(1):63–71. https://doi.org/10.14581/jer.21009.

Stephen LJ, Harden C, Tomson T, et al. Management of epilepsy in women. Lancet Neurol. 2019;18(5):481–91. https://doi.org/10.1016/S1474-4422(18)30495-2.

Thome-Souza S, Kuczynski E, Assumpção F, et al. Which factors may play a pivotal role on determining the type of psychiatric disorder in children and adolescents with epilepsy? Epilepsy Behav. 2004;5(6):988–94. https://doi.org/10.1016/j.yebeh.2004.09.001.

Tomson T, Battino D, Bonizzoni E, Craig J, Lindhout D, Perucca E, Sabers A, Thomas SV, Vajda F, EURAP Study Group. Comparative risk of major congenital malformations with eight different antiepileptic drugs: a prospective cohort study of the EURAP registry. Lancet Neurol. 2018;17(6):530–8. https://doi.org/10.1016/S1474-4422(18)30107-8.

Vajda FJE, O'Brien TJ, Graham JE, Hitchcock AA, Perucca P, Lander CM, Eadie MJ. Epileptic seizure control during and after pregnancy in Australian women. Acta Neurol Scand. 2022;145(6):730–6. https://doi.org/10.1111/ane.13609.

Vélez-Ruiz NJ, Pennell PB. Issues for women with epilepsy. Neurol Clin. 2016;34(2):411–25, ix. https://doi.org/10.1016/j.ncl.2015.11.009.

von Gaudecker JR, Taylor AG, Keeling AW, et al. Living in the epilepsy treatment gap in rural South India: a focused ethnography of women and problems associated with stigma. Health Care Women Int. 2017;38(7):753–64. https://doi.org/10.1080/07399332.2017.1321000.

Westbrook LE, Bauman LJ, Shinnar S. Applying stigma theory to epilepsy: a test of a conceptual model. J Pediatr Psychol. 1992;17(5):633–49. https://doi.org/10.1093/jpepsy/17.5.633.

Zupanc ML, Haut S. Epilepsy in women: special considerations for adolescents. Int Rev Neurobiol. 2008;83:91–111. https://doi.org/10.1016/S0074-7742(08)00005-6.

Suggested Readings

Albaghdadi O, Alhalabi MS, Alourfi Z, et al. Bone health and vitamin D status in young epilepsy patients on valproate monotherapy. Clin Neurol Neurosurg. 2016;146:52–6. https://doi.org/10.1016/j.clineuro.2016.04.019.

Ashwin M, Rakesh P, Pricilla RA, et al. Determinants of quality of life among people with epilepsy attending a secondary care rural hospital in South India. J Neurosci Rural Pract. 2013;4(Suppl 1):S62–6. https://doi.org/10.4103/0976-3147.116467.

Bangar S, Shastri A, El-Sayeh H, et al. Women with epilepsy: clinically relevant issues. Funct Neurol. 2016;31(3):127–34. https://doi.org/10.11138/fneur/2016.31.3.127.

Beerhorst K, van der Kruijs SJM, Verschuure P, et al. Bone disease during chronic antiepileptic drug therapy: general versus specific risk factors. J Neurol Sci. 2013;331(1–2):19–25. https://doi.org/10.1016/j.jns.2013.05.005.

Begum S, Thomas SV. Women with epilepsy in reproductive age group: special issues and management strategies. J Assoc Physicians India. 2013;61(8 Suppl):48–51.

Benavente-Aguilar I, Morales-Blánquez C, Rubio EA, et al. Quality of life of adolescents suffering from epilepsy living in the community. J Paediatr Child Health. 2004;40(3):110–3. https://doi.org/10.1111/j.1440-1754.2004.00308.x.

Burke EA, McCallion P, Carroll R, et al. An exploration of the bone health of older adults with an intellectual disability in Ireland. J Intellect Disabil Res. 2017;61(2):99–114. https://doi.org/10.1111/jir.12273.

Chaka A, Awoke T, Yohannis Z, et al. Determinants of depression among people with epilepsy in Central Ethiopia. Ann General Psychiatry. 2018;17:27. https://doi.org/10.1186/s12991-018-0197-z.

Danielsson KC, Borthen I, Morken NH, et al. Hypertensive pregnancy complications in women with epilepsy and antiepileptic drugs: a population-based cohort study of first pregnancies in Norway. BMJ Open. 2018;8(4):e020998. https://doi.org/10.1136/bmjopen-2017-020998.

Fraser LA, Burneo JG, Fraser JA. Enzyme-inducing antiepileptic drugs and fractures in people with epilepsy: a systematic review. Epilepsy Res. 2015;116:59–66. https://doi.org/10.1016/j.eplepsyres.2015.07.003.

Gil-Nagel A, López-Muñoz F, Serratosa JM, et al. Effect of lamotrigine on sexual function in patients with epilepsy. Seizure. 2006;15(3):142–9. https://pubmed.ncbi.nlm.nih.gov/16434217/.

Harden CL. Sexual dysfunction in women with epilepsy. Seizure. 2008;17(2):131–5. https://doi.org/10.1016/j.seizure.2007.11.010.

Harden CL, Pennell PB. Neuroendocrine considerations in the treatment of men and women with epilepsy. Lancet Neurol. 2013;12(1):72–83. https://doi.org/10.1016/S1474-4422(12)70239-9.

Hernández-Díaz S, McElrath TF, Pennell PB, et al. Fetal growth and premature delivery in pregnant women on antiepileptic drugs. Ann Neurol. 2017;82(3):457–65. https://doi.org/10.1002/ana.25031.

Kolstad E, Veiby G, Gilhus NE, et al. Overweight in epilepsy as a risk factor for pregnancy and delivery complications. Epilepsia. 2016;57(11):1849–57. https://doi.org/10.1111/epi.13573.

Koppel BS, Harden CL. Gender issues in the neurobiology of epilepsy: a clinical perspective. Neurobiol Dis. 2014;72 Pt B:193–7. https://doi.org/10.1016/j.nbd.2014.08.033.

Lee GH, Lee SA, No SK, et al. Factors contributing to the development of perceived stigma in people with newly diagnosed epilepsy: a one-year longitudinal study. Epilepsy Behav. 2016;54:1–6. https://doi.org/10.1016/j.yebeh.2015.10.024.

Lossius MI, Taubøll E, Mowinckel P, et al. Reversible effects of antiepileptic drugs on reproductive endocrine function in men and women with epilepsy—a prospective randomized double-blind withdrawal study. Epilepsia. 2007;48(10):1875–82. https://pubmed.ncbi.nlm.nih.gov/17555526/.

Margolis SA, Nakhutina L, Schaffer SG, et al. Perceived epilepsy stigma mediates relationships between personality and social well-being in a diverse epilepsy population. Epilepsy Behav. 2018;78:7–13. https://doi.org/10.1016/j.yebeh.2017.10.023.

Morrell MJ. Effects of epilepsy on women's reproductive health. Epilepsia. 1998;39(Suppl 8):S32–7. https://doi.org/10.1111/j.1528-1157.1998.tb02605.x.

Mostacci B, Bisulli F, Poluzzi E, et al. Emilia-Romagna Study on Pregnancy and Exposure to Antiepileptic drugs (ESPEA): a population-based study on prescription patterns, pregnancy outcomes and fetal health. J Neurol Neurosurg Psychiatry. 2018;89(9):983–8. https://doi.org/10.1136/jnnp-2017-317833.

Murthy RS. National Mental Health Survey of India 2015–2016. Indian J Psychiatry. 2017;59(1):21–6. https://doi.org/10.4103/psychiatry.IndianJPsychiatry_102_17.

Nicholas JM, Ridsdale L, Richardson MP, et al. Fracture risk with use of liver enzyme inducing antiepileptic drugs in people with active epilepsy: cohort study using the general practice research database. Seizure. 2013;22(1):37–42. https://doi.org/10.1016/j.seizure.2012.10.002.

Reimers A. Hormone replacement therapy with estrogens may reduce lamotrigine serum concentrations: a matched case-control study. Epilepsia. 2017;58(1):e6–9. https://doi.org/10.1111/epi.13597.

Reiter SF, Veiby G, Daltveit AK, et al. Psychiatric comorbidity and social aspects in pregnant women with epilepsy—the Norwegian Mother and Child Cohort Study. Epilepsy Behav. 2013;29(2):379–85. https://doi.org/10.1016/j.yebeh.2013.08.016.

Riasi H, Rajabpour Sanati A, Ghaemi K. The stigma of epilepsy and its effects on marital status. Springerplus. 2014;3:762. https://doi.org/10.1186/2193-1801-3-762.

Surís JC, Parera N, Puig C. Chronic illness and emotional distress in adolescence. J Adolesc Health. 1996;19(2):153–6. https://doi.org/10.1016/1054-139X(95)00231-G.

Verrotti A, Mencaroni E, Cofini M, et al. Valproic acid metabolism and its consequences on sexual functions. Curr Drug Metab. 2016;17(6):573–81. https://doi.org/10.2174/1389200217666160322143504.

Yeni K, Tulek Z, Simsek OF, et al. Relationships between knowledge, attitudes, stigma, anxiety and depression, and quality of life in epilepsy: a structural equation modeling. Epilepsy Behav. 2018;85:212–7. https://doi.org/10.1016/j.yebeh.2018.06.019.

Zhang YX, Shen CH, Lai QL, et al. Effects of antiepileptic drug on thyroid hormones in patients with epilepsy: a meta-analysis. Seizure. 2016;35:72–9. https://doi.org/10.1016/j.seizure.2016.01.010.

Diagnosis and Treatment of Women with Epilepsy

2

Ziyi Chen, Xinling Geng, Yulong Li, Leihao Sha, Yutong Fu, and Lei Chen

2.1 Advances in the Diagnosis and Treatment of Epilepsy

Ziyi Chen, Xinling Geng, and Leihao Sha

2.1.1 Epilepsy: Related Definitions and Diagnostic Criteria

In 2014, the International League Against Epilepsy (ILAE) defined epilepsy as a brain disorder that meets any of the following conditions: (1) at least two unprovoked (or reflexive) seizures >24 h apart, (2) having one unprovoked (or reflexive) seizure with a probability of having another seizure within the next 10 years similar to the risk of recurrence after two unprovoked seizures (at least 60%), and (3) a diagnosis of epileptic syndrome. The following conditions are considered to define a seizure-free state: (1) age-related seizure syndrome but now past the appropriate age for seizures and (2) no seizures in the past 10 years as well as no antiseizure medications in the past 5 years. In 2015, the Chinese Antiepileptic Association also revised the clinical diagnosis and treatment guidelines for epilepsy, defining epilepsy not as a single disease entity but as a chronic brain disease state with different

Z. Chen
Department of Neurology, The First Affiliated Hospital, Sun Yat-sen University, Guangzhou, China
e-mail: chenziyi@mail.sysu.edu.cn

X. Geng
School of Biomedical Engineering, Capital Medical University, Beijing, China
e-mail: gengxl@ccmu.edu.cn

Y. Li · L. Sha · Y. Fu · L. Chen (✉)
Department of Neurology, West China Hospital, Sichuan University, Chengdu, China

L. Chen (ed.), *Women with Epilepsy in Child-bearing Age*,
https://doi.org/10.1007/978-981-97-3921-9_2

etiologies and clinical manifestations, but with repeated seizures as a common feature.

Epilepsy that cannot be controlled after standardized drug use is called drug-resistant epilepsy. In 2010, the ILAE proposed diagnostic criteria for drug-resistant epilepsy, as follows: the correct selection of two tolerable antiseizure medications that, after enough courses and doses of a single drug or combined treatment, fail to result in seizure freedom. The criteria also specify that the seizure-free period must be three times as long as the maximum interval between seizures before treatment or 1 year (whichever is longer). The definition has been widely used, but at present, many areas in China still apply the standard of drug tolerance epilepsy proposed by domestic scholars: the application of appropriate and regular ASM treatment and a drug concentration within the effective range, frequent seizures (at least 4 or more times per month), seizures observed for more than 2 years, uncontrolled seizures that affect the patient's quality of life; and the exclusion of intracranial space occupying lesion(s) and/or progressive central nervous system disease.

Status epilepticus (SE) is an acute and critical condition encountered in neurology departments. The emergence of SE is associated with a significant increase in the disability rate and fatality rate among patients with epilepsy. The edition of the ILAE guidelines published in 2015 provided a new definition and classification of SE, whereby SE is defined as the failure of a mechanism that terminates seizures or a new epileptogenic mechanism that leads to an unusually durable epileptic seizure (t_1) and may cause long-term damage (t_2), resulting in more serious consequences including neuronal damage or even death, and changes in the structure of neural networks. Regarding the t_1 and t_2 time concepts and thresholds: (1) for tonic-clonic seizures, t_1 is 5 min and t_2 is 30 min; (2) for focal seizures with impaired consciousness, t_1 is 10 min and t_2 is >60 min; and (3) for absence seizures, t_1 is 10–15 min and t_2 is undetermined. SE can be classified by seizure type into convulsive SE and non-convulsive SE, with the former being the commonest. In 2017, the ILAE revised the classification of seizures and epilepsy, and classified epileptic seizures into three categories: focal origin, general origin, and unknown origin; simultaneously, the causes of epilepsy were also newly classified into genetic, structural, infectious, immune, metabolic, and unknown etiology, which is more suitable for clinical application.

2.1.2 Treatment of Epilepsy

Early recognition and early diagnosis of epilepsy is the key to the reasonable selection of treatment and improvement of patient prognosis. At present, epilepsy treatment mainly comprises drug therapy, neurostimulation treatment, surgery, ketogenic diet, and stem cell therapy.

2.1.2.1 Drug Therapy

Currently, ASMs remain the mainstay of epilepsy treatment, and approximately 70% of newly diagnosed epilepsy patients can attain seizure control by taking a single ASM; thus, the initial drug selection process is very important, as correct drug selection can increase treatment success. According to the type of seizure, etiology, and syndrome classification, drug selection is the basic principle of epilepsy treatment. Other factors to be considered include contraindications, adverse reactions, time to reach the therapeutic dose, the number of daily administrations and appropriate dosage form, special populations (including children, women of childbearing age, and the elderly), drug interactions, drug sources, and drug costs.

If seizures cannot be controlled, the treatment options include one of the following three. The first option is to increase the ASM dose, but single-drug treatment is prone to lead to drug resistance and reduce the effective concentration of drugs. Although increasing the dose of ASMs can improve the concentration of drugs in the brain, the associated side effects are also large and this option is not recommended for long-term use. The second option is the use of new ASMs. The advent of new ASMs provides the possibility for effective treatment of refractory epilepsy, and the treatment can be remarkable. The third option is the combined application of ASMs. According to the patient's condition, adjustment of the drug doses and ratios can have good effects and result in strong targeted treatment. When choosing the drugs to combine, ASMs with different mechanisms of action should be selected; in addition, drugs with the same side effects and complex interactions should be avoided, and blood drug concentrations should be regularly monitored to adjust the medication dosages accordingly.

2.1.2.2 Surgical Treatment

With the continuous improvement of preoperative evaluation methods, the surgical treatment of refractory epilepsy has been greatly advanced. Preoperative surgical evaluation methods include non-invasive and invasive techniques, non-invasive examinations include clinical symptomatologic assessment, electroencephalogram (EEG), magnetoencephalogram (MEG), magnetic resonance imaging (MRI), single photon emission computed tomography (SPECT), and positron emission tomography (PET). Invasive monitoring methods include subdural electrode implantation to monitor EEG, cortical electroencephalography (ECoG), and intracranial deep electrode EEG. At present, the commonly used surgical methods are divided into curative and palliative operations, the former including focal resection and hemispherectomy, while the latter includes corpus callosotomy and multiple subpial transections. Surgical procedures are used to control epilepsy by removing the epileptogenic focus, destroying the excitatory structure(s), cutting off the discharge pathway, or stimulating inhibitory structures. With the continuous development of microneurosurgical techniques, the incidence of refractory epilepsy has been reduced and the disability rate has been gradually reduced.

2.1.2.3 Ketogenic Diet Therapy

Ketogenic diet therapy has been used for epilepsy treatment for over a century, and involves placing patients with epilepsy on a diet high in fat, low in protein, and low in carbohydrates to induce a state of ketosis that mimics starvation and thus inhibits seizures. It was first used in children under the age of 12 because their brains have a better ability to take up and use ketogenic bodies than adults. However, some recent studies have suggested that the ketogenic diet may have some effect on drug-resistant epilepsy in adolescents and adults as well. Although the efficacy of the ketogenic diet has long been recognized, it is associated with a variety of adverse reactions affecting the major systems of the human body, and the compliance of patients can be poor. Possible adverse reactions include hypertriglyceridemia, hypercholesterolemia, increased uric acid levels, various infectious diseases, hypoglycemia, hypoproteinemia, and electrolyte disorders. Therefore, the treatment should be strictly standardized, and its safety, applicability, and compliance need to be improved.

2.1.2.4 Neurostimulation Treatment

2.1.2.4.1 Vagus Nerve Stimulation

Vagus nerve stimulation (VNS) is a well-established method for treating drug-resistant epilepsy. By implanting a small device that delivers electrical impulses to the vagus nerve, VNS has shown a promising ability to modulate neural activities within the brain, thereby reducing seizure frequency in a significant portion of patients. Since its FDA approval in 1997, VNS has been shown to reduce seizure frequency by at least 50% in approximately 50–60% of patients who do not respond to antiseizure medications. The mechanism by which VNS exerts its antiepileptic effects is not fully understood. It's hypothesized that changes in neurotransmitter levels and the modulation of brain networks play crucial roles. The treatment, while effective, is not devoid of side effects such as hoarseness, cough, and throat pain. Nevertheless, the sustained seizure frequency reduction and quality of life improvements render VNS an invaluable option for those grappling with refractory epilepsy.

2.1.2.4.2 Deep Brain Stimulation

Deep brain stimulation (DBS) for epilepsy involves the surgical implantation of electrodes in specific brain regions associated with seizure activity, notably the anterior nucleus of the thalamus (ANT), to deliver electrical pulses aimed at interrupting seizure propagation pathways. Approved by the FDA in 2018 for drug-resistant epilepsy, DBS has been reported to reduce seizure frequency by approximately 40–60% for those inadequately managed by medications. Although the exact mechanism remains under study, it is believed that DBS's efficacy stems from its ability to modulate the thalamocortical circuits, which is essential in the generation and spread of seizures. As a reversible and adjustable seizure control method, DBS stands as a beacon of hope, albeit with its share of risks including infection and hemorrhage, underscoring the need for meticulous patient selection.

2.1.2.4.3 Responsive Neurostimulation

Responsive neurostimulation (RNS) marks a significant advancement in the neurostimulation treatment for epilepsy. The RNS system, consisting of a neurostimulator implanted within the cranium and connected to leads positioned at the seizure focus, represents a targeted approach to seizure management. This system is designed to monitor brain activity continuously, identifying abnormal electrical patterns indicative of an impending seizure and intervening with precise electrical stimulation to prevent it. The efficacy of RNS in reducing seizure frequency in drug-resistant focal epilepsy has been substantiated through clinical trials, offering a favorable safety profile predominantly associated with the implantation process rather than the stimulation itself. The exact mechanisms through which RNS exerts its effects are still under investigation but are believed to involve the modulation of epileptogenic networks, restoration of normal neuronal activity, and possibly, long-term plasticity changes within the brain. The exploration of RNS's mechanisms and optimization of stimulation parameters heralds an era of more effective, potentially less invasive treatments for a broader patient demographic.

2.1.2.4.4 tDCS/tACS

Transcranial direct/alternating current Stimulation (tDCS) is promising non-invasive brain stimulation techniques that have garnered attention for their potential in treating epilepsy. By applying electrical currents to the scalp, these methods seek to modify abnormal neural activity underlying epilepsy. The allure of tDCS and tACS lies in their potential to directly target brain areas implicated in seizure initiation and propagation without surgical intervention, offering a patient-friendly treatment option. By modulating the cortical excitability, these techniques aim to reduce the frequency and intensity of seizures in individuals with drug-resistant epilepsy. Preliminary studies have suggested that tDCS can decrease seizure occurrence and improve cognitive outcomes in some patients. Similarly, tACS, particularly at frequencies that disrupt pathological brain rhythms, has shown potential in reducing epileptiform activity. The mechanisms underlying the antiepileptic effects of tDCS and tACS are believed to involve the normalization of neuronal firing rates and the restoration of functional connectivity within brain networks disrupted by epilepsy. Despite their potential, the application of tDCS and tACS in epilepsy treatment faces several challenges, including determining the optimal stimulation parameters (such as intensity, duration, and frequency), identifying the most effective stimulation sites, and understanding individual variability in response to treatment. Future research will need to address these issues through carefully designed clinical trials, aiming to establish standardized protocols that maximize the efficacy and safety of tDCS and tACS for epilepsy patients. Moreover, combining these stimulation techniques with other treatments, such as pharmacotherapy or behavioral interventions, may enhance their therapeutic benefits.

2.1.2.4.5 Transcranial Magnetic Stimulation for Epilepsy

Transcranial magnetic stimulation (TMS) is another non-invasive technique that uses magnetic fields to induce electrical currents in specific brain regions. TMS has been explored for its therapeutic potential in epilepsy, with studies indicating that repetitive TMS (rTMS) can lead to a significant reduction in seizure frequency and an improvement in quality of life, presumably through the modulation of cortical excitability and synaptic plasticity. These alterations in brain communication and network dynamics might underlie the mechanism of seizure generation. While promising, the clinical application of TMS in epilepsy requires further elucidation of optimal stimulation parameters, target regions, and session frequencies to maximize therapeutic outcomes. Moreover, TMS's effects appear to be transient, highlighting the necessity of a sustained treatment regimen to maintain seizure reduction. Ongoing research aims to refine TMS protocols and understand its mechanism to enhance its efficacy as a treatment for drug-resistant epilepsy.

2.1.2.4.6 Ultrasound Stimulation

Ultrasound stimulation (US), particularly focused ultrasound (FUS) offers a non-invasive approach to modulating brain activity and potentially reducing seizure frequency, represents an emerging frontier in the treatment of epilepsy. Distinct from traditional neurostimulation techniques, FUS employs high-frequency sound waves to precisely target brain regions involved in seizures. This method's precision and non-surgical nature significantly reduce patient discomfort and infection risk. Recent studies have begun to explore the efficacy and safety of FUS in animal models and limited human trials, showing promising results in reducing seizure occurrence and severity. The mechanism behind FUS's antiepileptic effects is believed to involve the temporary alteration of cell membrane permeability and the modulation of local and network-wide brain activity, thereby disrupting the pathological synchrony that underlies epileptic seizures. Additionally, FUS has the potential to open the blood–brain barrier (BBB) in a controlled manner, which could facilitate the delivery of therapeutic agents directly to seizure foci, further enhancing its antiepileptic effects. Despite its potential, the application of FUS in epilepsy treatment is still in its infancy, with numerous challenges to overcome. These include optimizing ultrasound parameters for maximal efficacy, ensuring safety, particularly with repeated applications, and determining the long-term effects of such treatment. Future research directions will likely focus on refining FUS technology, expanding clinical trials to a broader range of epilepsy patients, and exploring combinatory therapies that leverage FUS's unique capabilities.

2.1.2.4.7 Sensory Stimulation for Epilepsy

Sensory stimulation as a therapeutic approach for epilepsy is based on the premise that certain sensory inputs can influence brain activity and potentially modulate seizure occurrence. This can include auditory, visual, or tactile stimulation. Recent research has explored the use of specific types of sensory stimulation, such as auditory or visual stimuli, to reduce seizure frequency or severity in individuals with epilepsy. Recent studies have explored the use of auditory stimulation during sleep to suppress epileptiform activity, particularly in syndromes like benign epilepsy with centrotemporal spikes. This method's non-invasiveness and ease of implementation make it an attractive option, potentially even for home use. Despite its promise, the effectiveness of sensory stimulation in epilepsy treatment remains highly variable, contingent upon the stimulation type, frequency, and timing relative to seizure activity, alongside individual sensory processing differences. Future investigations aim to unravel optimal stimulation protocols, integrating sensory stimulation with other treatments to forge a comprehensive epilepsy management strategy.

2.1.2.4.8 Future Directions

The landscape of neurostimulation therapies for epilepsy is characterized by rapid advancements, offering renewed hope for individuals with drug-resistant epilepsy. From invasive techniques like VNS, DBS, and RNS to non-invasive approaches such as tDCS/tACS, TMS, US and sensory stimulation, each modality presents unique benefits and challenges. Ongoing research endeavors to refine treatment protocols, identify suitable patient populations, and elucidate mechanisms of action. Future research will likely focus on identifying new stimulation targets, refining existing technologies to increase their precision and reduce invasiveness, and exploring the synergistic potential of combining different therapeutic modalities. With ongoing advancements, neurostimulation therapies are poised to become more accessible, less invasive, and more effective, offering new hope to millions of people living with drug-resistant epilepsy. This dynamic and evolving landscape underscores the critical importance of continued innovation, interdisciplinary collaboration, and patient-centered research in unlocking the full potential of neurostimulation in epilepsy treatment.

2.1.2.5 Stem Cell Therapy (Experimental Treatment)

Stem cell transplantation is the implantation of nerve tissue or a stem cell suspension into a patient's brain to repair or replace damaged or denatured nerve cells and restore the normal regulatory function of the brain. Theoretically, stem cell transplantation can replace damaged or excised neurons or secrete neurotrophic factors to promote the repair of damaged neurons. Stem cell transplantation has achieved some results in a large number of animal models. There are also successful cases in clinical studies, but the long-term effects and potential safety following treatment have not been elucidated, and thus it has not been widely used in clinical practice. With the continuous advances in science and technology, there are many prospects for the application of emerging technologies such as gene therapy and cell transplantation in refractory epilepsy.

2.2 Traditional Chinese Medicine Diagnosis and Treatment of Epilepsy

Yulong Li

2.2.1 The Historical Understanding of Epilepsy in Traditional Chinese Medicine

During the Spring and Autumn period and the Warring States period, the disease was initially called "*Dian Ji* (meaning the vertex disease)," recognized as a sort of "fetal illness." In the book "*SuWen-Qi Bing Lun(Plain Questions—On Extraordinary Diseases)*" it states: "Some people are born with epilepsy… the disease is called fetal illness. This is acquired when the mother is frightened during pregnancy, which causes the qi to rise and not descend, leading to the combination of essence and qi, and thus causing the child to develop epilepsy." In the book "*Ling Shu-Dian Kuang(Miraculous Pivot—Epilepsy)*," it mentions: "When epilepsy first occurs, there are initially tonic seizures and then progress to spinal spasm." It believes that the onset of the disease is related to congenital factors and also describes the clinical manifestations of muscle rigidity followed by spinal spasms during seizure episodes.

During the Sui and Tang dynasties, the terms "*Dian Chi*(Epilepsy)" or "*Xian*(Eclampsia)" were first proposed as names for the disease, with more specific records of the names and symptoms of epilepsy. Chao Yuanfang, in his work *Zhu Bing Yuan Hou Lun—Xian Hou* described the symptoms of the disease as follows: "Sometimes the mouth and eyes are drawn together, causing the eyes to shake; or there may be spasms in the hands and feet; or there may be rigidity in the back, or bending of the neck." He also classified the disease into different types based on different causes, such as "wind-induced epilepsy," "fright-induced epilepsy," and "food-induced epilepsy." In another work, *Zhu Bing Yuan Hou Lun—Xian Hou-Dian Kuang Hou*," it states: "Suddenly, the person falls down, foams at the mouth, shouts, eyes bulge, hands and feet are convulsed, and they have no consciousness. It takes a long time for them to regain their senses." The author provides a detailed description of the clinical symptoms of this disease. In *Zhu Bing Yuan Hou Lun—Wu Dian Bing Hou*, it points out that the disease has the characteristics of repeated attacks. Sun Simiao first introduced the term "epilepsy" and categorized its 20 different symptoms in his book *Bei Ji Qian Jin Yao Fang (Essential Prescriptions for Emergencies)*. In the same volume, the author underscores the significance of monitoring the psychological state preceding the onset of an epileptic seizure.

During the Song, Jin, and Yuan dynasties, there was a deeper understanding of the etiology and pathogenesis of the disease. Chen Yan, in his work *San Yin Ji Yi Bing Zheng Fang Lun—Dian Xian Xun Lun (Discussion on Epilepsy in 'Three Causes, Ultimate Unity' Theory)*, stated: "Epilepsy is caused by shock, which disrupts the balance of visceral qi, causing stagnation and the generation of saliva, blocking the meridians, and leading to sudden convulsions. It can be caused by shocks received in the mother's womb, exposure to external factors like wind, cold, heat, and dampness during childhood, or improper diet that goes against the flow of visceral qi." He pointed out that various factors such as fear, external influences of phlegm and saliva, and improper diet could lead to imbalances in visceral qi and disturb the balance between yin and yang, causing mental disorders and illness. Yan Yonghe, in his work *Ji Sheng Fang—Xian Xian Lun Zhi (Ji Sheng Fang: Discussion on the Treatment of Epilepsy)*, stated, "The classification of epilepsy aligns with the five zang-organs, which, in turn, correspond to five animals, thereby categorizing epilepsy based on the five zang-organs." Zhang Zihe, in his work *Ru Men Shi Qin—Volume 11*, stated, "Usually, when wind-induced epilepsy occurs, there is stiffness in the neck and eyes, and a loss of consciousness. This is due to heat in the liver meridian." Zhu Zhenheng, in his work "*Dan Xi Xin Fa—Xian (Dan Xi's Heart Method: Epilepsy)*," pointed out that the underlying cause of epilepsy is the obstruction of orifices by phlegm and fluid leading to confusion and delirium. He advocated focusing on resolving phlegm.

During the Ming and Qing dynasties, the theoretical understanding of the disease progressively improved. Gong Xin, in his book "Gu Jin Yi Jian·Wu Bing *(Ancient and Modern Medical Mirror)*": *Five Diseases*, believed that epilepsy is often caused by the stagnation of the seven emotions, external pathogenic factors, or fright, which lead to the unclear mind by phlegm. The treatment should focus on resolving phlegm, regulating qi, clearing heat, and harmonizing the liver. Wang Kentang, in his work "Treatment Principles and General Discussion on Disease Identification," differentiated between the three types of epilepsy and mania, marking a significant advancement in the understanding of these conditions. Cheng Guopen, in his book, *Yi Xue Xin Wu—Dian Kuang Xian (Medical Enlightenment: Mania and Epilepsy)*, created the Epilepsy Pill, the representative of herbal prescriptions used for epilepsy till today. Li Yongcui, in his work, *Zheng Zhi Hui Bu: Xian Bing (Compendium of Diagnosis and Treatment: Epilepsy)*, proposed differentiating between Yang Epilepsy and Yin Epilepsy and corresponding treatment principles based on the differentiation. Ye Tianshi, in his book, *Lin Zheng Zhi Nan Yi An—Dian Xian (Clinical Guide to Medical Records: Epilepsy)* stated, "For the excess type of epilepsy, Wuxian Pill could be used to address wind, Kongxian Pill to alleviate phlegm, and Longhui Pill to clear heat; for the deficiency type, focus on nourishing qi and blood, balancing yin and yang, and using Yingying Decoction and Heche Pill as the main treatments." The approach advocated considering both excess and deficiency patterns in the treatment of epilepsy. Wang Qingren, in his book *Yi Lin Gai Cuo—Bi Zheng You Yu Xue Shuo (Medical Forest Corrections: Theory of Blood Stasis in Paralysis)*, believed that the occurrence of epilepsy is related to "deficiency of vital qi" and "stagnation of blood in the brain and marrow." He developed the Longma Zilai Pill and Huangchi Feng Decoction for the treatment of epilepsy related to deficiency of qi with blood stasis, which is still valuable in the treatment today.

2.2.2 Insights on Epilepsy in Traditional Chinese Medicine

TCM believed the etiology of epilepsy can be categorized into two: congenital factors and acquired factors. Congenital factors primarily involve insufficient or abnormal innate endowment. Acquired factors include emotional disturbances, improper diet, falls or external injuries, or brain damage caused by other illnesses. Both can lead to dysfunction of the organs and obstruction of the mind by wind, heat, phlegm, and blood stasis. The accumulation of phlegm internally may be triggered by occasional causes, resulting in disharmony of viseral qi, imbalance of yin and yang, and the onset of the disease. Figure 2.1 showed the various diagnosis factors of epilepsy in TCM.

1. Abnormal innate endowment is often observed in the onset of epilepsy during childhood, which is closely related to congenital factors. As the saying goes, "epilepsy is due to insufficient prenatal yin essence." When the fetus is in the mother's womb, if the mother experiences a sudden fright, it can cause the reversal of qi circulation and injure the essence, resulting in kidney deficiency.

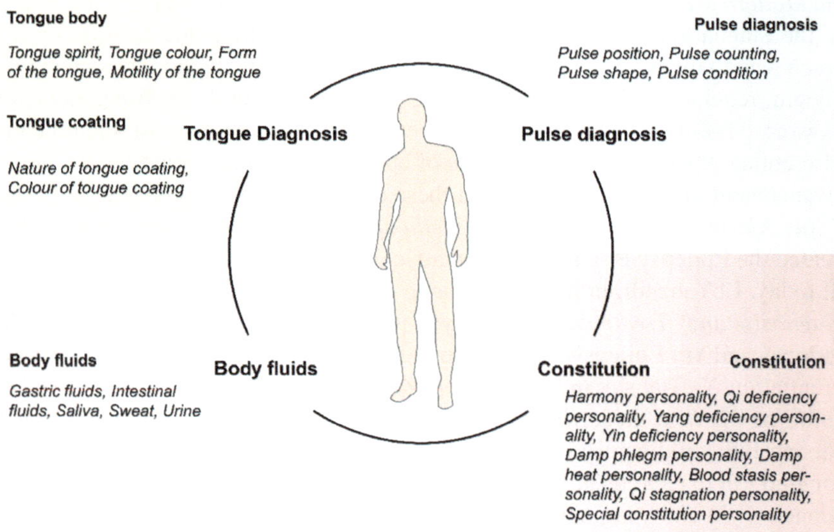

Fig. 2.1 Various diagnosis factors of epilepsy in TCM

Additionally, if the mother experiences multiple illnesses, excessive fatigue, or improper medication during pregnancy, it can harm the fetus and impair the fetal qi, leading to abnormal development after birth and the onset of this disease. Moreover, if either parent has weak constitutional strength leading to inadequate innate endowment in the fetus or if either parent has epilepsy causing disharmony in viseceral qi, it can result in abnormal innate endowment in the fetus, making it more susceptible to developing epilepsy.

2. Emotional imbalance: Among the Seven Emotions, the main cause lies in fear and fright. As mentioned in *Zheng Zhi Hui Bu—Xian Bing(Compendium of Diagnosis and Treatment: Epilepsy)*, it states: "Sometimes it occurs due to sudden fright. When frightened, the spirit departs, leaving an empty shell, and phlegm takes advantage of the opportunity to invade." Sudden fright can cause a disturbance in qi circulation, with phlegm and turbidity ascending against the flow of qi, obstructing the clear orifices. Excessive emotional stimulation or long-standing liver depression transforming into fire can lead to the invasion of wind and fire together with phlegm, disrupting the control of the primordial spirit and resulting in the disease. Children have delicate organs and insufficient vital qi. Their spirit and qi are fragile, making them more prone to panic and developing the disease.
3. Improper diet: Overeating fatty, sweet, and greasy food can damage the spleen and stomach, impairing their healthy function and causing the accumulation of

dampness and the formation of phlegm. Alternatively, if qi stagnation transforms into fire, the pathogenic fire can evaporate fluids and form phlegm, leading to the accumulation of hidden phlegm. When triggered by certain factors, the turbid phlegm can obscure the clear orifices of the primordial spirit, resulting in this disease.

4. Brain damage: Brain injuries caused by falls, collisions, dystocia, or other illnesses such as intracranial infections or poisoning can lead to stagnation and obstruction of cerebral blood vessels or damage to the brain orifices. This can result in a disturbance of consciousness, confusion, and ignorance, leading to the onset of this disease.

This disease primarily resides in the brain and is closely related to the heart, liver, spleen, and kidneys. The basic pathological mechanism involves the accumulation of hidden phlegm, which is triggered by wind and fire. The interaction between phlegm and stasis leads to obstruction, resulting in the obscuration of the clear orifices and the onset of the disease. As mentioned in *Yi Xue Gang Mu—Dian Xian (Medical Principles: Epilepsy)*, it states: "Epilepsy is caused by the reverse ascent of pathogenic phlegm." The disease primarily affects the brain and is closely associated with the heart, liver, spleen, and kidneys. The pathological factors involve wind, fire, phlegm, stasis, among which the dominance of pathogenic phlegm is particularly important. The phlegm in epilepsy has two characteristics: it tends to gather or disperse with the movement of wind and cannot be easily transformed. When phlegm accumulates and qi rises against its natural flow, it obstructs the clear orifices, leading to epilepsy episodes. When the phlegm descends and qi flows smoothly, the episodes subside. If wind, yang, phlegm, and fire rise and do not descend, then major seizures may occur. The duration and interval of the episodes are closely related to the smooth or obstructed flow of qi and the degree of phlegm stagnation. Due to the stubbornness and difficulty in transforming the phlegm, epilepsy can persist for a long time and may recur repeatedly.

The pathological nature of this disease is a combination of deficiency and excess. In the early stages, the predominant manifestation is excess, characterized by wind-phlegm obstruction, phlegm-fire obstructing the orifices, or the intermingling of phlegm and stasis. In the later stages, due to the prolonged progression of the disease and damage to the body's vital qi, the condition often presents a mixture of deficiency and excess. Onset of epilepsy in childhood is often associated with inherent deficiencies, with the disease predominantly being a combination of deficiency and mild excess. During the seizure phase, the condition is mostly characterized by excess or a combination of excess and deficiency, while the remission phase is mostly characterized by deficiency or a combination of deficiency and excess. The remission phase is only a temporary relief of the pathogenic factors such as wind, fire, phlegm, and stasis. However, since the underlying cause has not been eliminated, residual phlegm remains, and organ function fails to fully recover, a relapse can occur at any time. The transformation of the pathological mechanism of this disease depends on the strength or weakness of the body's vital energy and the depth of the phlegm pathology. In the early stages of the disease, when phlegm and stasis obstruct the orifices, liver depression transforms into fire, which gives rise to wind. Due to the relatively abundant vital qi and superficially located phlegm and stagnant blood, the recovery is more likely. However, if the condition persists without improvement, phlegm and stasis can become solidified and obstructive, resulting in damage to the vital qi, leading to a mixture of deficiency and excess. The deep-seated phlegm becomes difficult to eliminate, making treatment more challenging. As this disease often fluctuates between active and remission phases, and tends to recur, if left untreated for a long time, it will further weaken the organs and deepen the phlegm pathology, resulting in stubborn phlegm. When stubborn phlegm is difficult to eliminate, epilepsy episodes recur, leading to a chronic condition.

2.2.3 TCM Syndrome Differentiation and Treatment of Epilepsy

2.2.3.1 Epileptic Phase

1. Yang Eclampsia

Clinical presentation: Sudden collapse, unconsciousness, facial flushing or purple-red complexion, followed by cyanosis or pallor, cyanotic lips, clenched jaws, upward gaze, stiff neck and back, convulsions of limbs, drooling or phlegm rattling in the throat, or bizarre cries, and in severe cases, involuntary urination and defecation, with eventual awakening after a period. Prior to the onset, there are often premonitory symptoms such as dizziness, headache with a feeling of pressure, chest tightness and weakness, frequent yawning; emotionally, there is often irritability, restlessness, insomnia, bitter taste in the mouth, dry throat, constipation, and dark urine; the tongue is red with a white greasy or yellow greasy coating, and the pulse is wiry and rapid or slippery and rapid.

Treatment principle: Urgently open the orifices and awaken the spirit, followed by clearing heat, eliminating phlegm, and calming the wind.

2. Yin Epilepsy

Clinical manifestations: Sudden collapse, unconsciousness, dull and grayish-yellow complexion, coldness in the extremities, semi-closed eyes, rigid limbs, or twitching movements, foaming at the mouth, generally no crying or only faint vocalizations, feelings of exhaustion throughout the body upon awakening, or normal functioning. Alternatively, it may present as transient dazedness, unawareness, unresponsiveness, immobility, and muteness, lasting from a few seconds to several minutes before recovery. After recovery, there is no recollection of the aforementioned symptoms. It may occur several times a day or even dozens of times. Common symptoms include fatigue, weakness, nausea, vomiting, chest tightness, cough with phlegm, poor appetite, and loose stools. The tongue appears pale with a white greasy coating, and the pulse is usually deep, thin, or delayed.

Treatment principles: Urgently open the orifices to restore consciousness, then resolve phlegm and saliva with warmth, regulate qi, and stabilize seizures.

Prescription: Wu Sheng Fluid combined with Er Chen Decoction.

2.2.3.2 Epileptic Interval

1. Liver Fire and Phlegm-Heat

Clinical manifestations: Usually irritable and easily angered, red face and eyes, restlessness and insomnia, uncomfortable cough with phlegm, bitter taste and dry throat, constipation, and dark yellow urine. During a flare-up, there may be unconsciousness, seizures, excessive saliva, or yelling. The tongue is red with a yellow greasy coating, and the pulse is wiry, slippery, and rapid.

Treatment principles: Clear the liver, relieve fire, transform phlegm, and calm the mind.

Representative prescription: Long Dan Xie Gan Decoction combined with Di Tan Decoction.

2. Spleen Deficiency and Phlegm Excess

Clinical manifestations: Chronic fatigue, lack of energy, lazy speech, stuffiness and oppression in the chest and epigastric region, poor appetite, and loose stools. During a flare-up, the complexion may appear dull or pale, limbs feel cool, curled-up position with rigidity, vomiting saliva, and low timid voice. The tongue appears pale with a white greasy coating, and the pulse is slippery or thin and slippery.

Treatment principles: Strengthen the spleen and transform phlegm.

Representative prescription: Liu Jun Zi Decoction.

3. Liver and Kidney Yin Deficiency

Clinical manifestations: Frequent seizures, confusion, dull complexion, dizziness, accompanied by dry and gritty eyes, withered and dull earlobes, forgetfulness, insomnia, sore and weak lower back and knees, and dry stools. The tongue is red with a thin white or thin yellow coating and scanty fluids, and the pulse is deep, thin, and rapid.

Treatment principles: Nourish the liver and kidney, replenish essence, and nourish the marrow.

Representative prescription: Da Bu Yuan Jian.

4. Blood Stasis Blocking Brain Collaterals

Clinical manifestations: Chronic dizziness, epileptic seizures with fixed location, often accompanied by unilateral limb convulsions or facial twitching, cyanosis or purplish discoloration of the face and lips. The tongue appears dark red or with ecchymosis, thin white coating, and the pulse is choppy or wiry. It often occurs after stroke, cranial trauma, childbirth-related injury, or intracranial infectious diseases.

Treatment principles: Activate blood circulation, dissolve blood stasis, relieve wind, and open collaterals.

Representative prescription: Tong Qiao Huo Xue Decoction.

2.2.4 Progress of TCM Research in Epilepsy

1. Acupuncture Treatment (Fig. 2.2)

The general principles of acupuncture treatment for epilepsy are consistent with medication treatment, that is, to treat the symptoms when they occur and address the root causes in the long term. According to the treatment principles, acupuncture points along the Du meridian are often selected in clinical practice for epilepsy treatment. The combination of acupuncture points is also determined based on syndrome differentiation and treatment, which may include points from the Spleen, Heart, Liver, Kidney, and other meridians. Commonly used acupuncture points include *Zhongwan, Qihai, Guanyuan, Zusanli, Fenglong, Sanyinjiao, Taichong*, and *Qiu Xu*, among others.

In addition, acupuncture can improve the pathological changes in the hippocampus. The mechanism of acupuncture treatment for epilepsy may be related to local stimulation inhibiting the expression of nuclear transcription factor-kappa B (NF-κB) in hippocampal nerve cells, weakening the acute inflammatory process involving NF-κB, inhibiting inflammatory factors, reducing apoptosis of normal hippocampal nerve cells, and thus reducing the frequency and duration of epileptic seizures and alleviating epileptic symptoms. Acupuncture treatment has a beneficial and multi-directional regulatory effect. It not only alleviates symptoms, improves the effectiveness of antiepileptic treatment, and reduces the incidence of complications but also regulates the functions of various organs. Currently, acupuncture treatment for epilepsy has been widely used in clinical practice, and most reports indicate reliable treatment efficacy, indicating that acupuncture treatment for epilepsy has certain advantages and potential for further development.

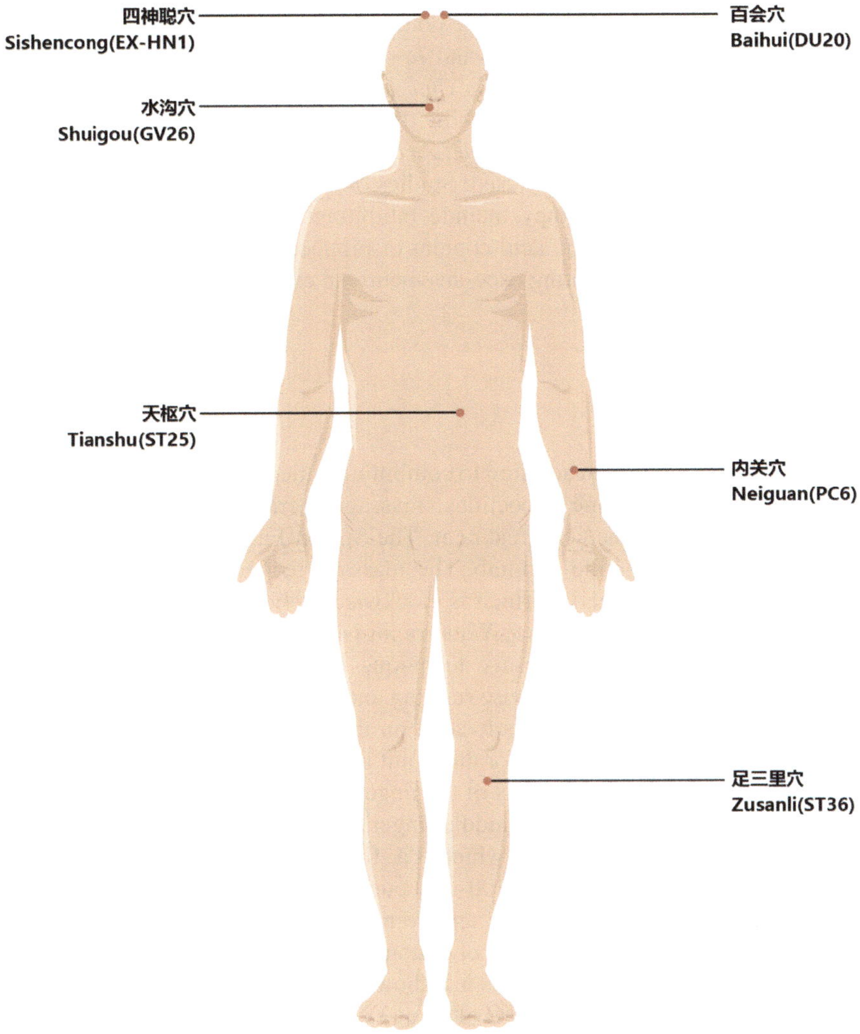

Fig. 2.2 Acupuncture treatment of epilepsy in TCM

2. Acupoint Catenary Treatment
Catgut embedding therapy is a type of external treatment in traditional Chinese medicine. Due to its ease of implementation, long-lasting effects, and good compliance, it is often combined with western medicine for the treatment of epilepsy. The catgut is embedded on acupoints once every week, with a different group of acupuncture points selected each time.

The commonly used acupuncture points for thread embedding therapy for epilepsy are as follows: *Fenglong* and *Taichong* are often selected for resolving phlegm and calming wind; *Xin Chu* and *Gan Shu* are commonly chosen for regulating the five organs, soothing the liver, and consolidating the mind. Additionally, *Dazhui, Jinshu, Jiuwei, Zusanli, Binao, Baihui, Yaoji*, and other acupoints are also commonly used. Studies have shown that the mechanisms of catgut embedding therapy include inhibiting apoptosis of hippocampal cells, regulating the amino acid content of hippocampal neurons, regulating brain cell function, inhibiting excessive neuronal excitability, and modulating brain wave frequencies.

3. *Tuina* Therapy

For pediatric epilepsy, in addition to combining antiepileptic drugs with traditional Chinese medicine decoctions, massage therapy can be used as an adjunctive Chinese medical treatment. The Spleen Earth point is located on the fingertip of the child's thumb. The massage technique for this point is tonifying the Spleen Earth, which is clockwise rubbing and kneading of the Spleen Earth point. The Kidney Water point is located on the fingertip of the child's little finger. The massage technique for this point is tonifying the Kidney Water, which is clockwise rubbing and kneading of the Kidney Water point. The Liver Wood point is located on the fingertip of the child's index finger. The massage technique for this point is clearing the Liver Wood, which is a straight push toward the root of the finger. The Heart Fire point is located on the fingertip of the child's middle finger. The massage technique for this point is clearing the Heart Fire, which is a straight push toward the root of the finger. For each point, perform 200–300 pushes or kneads in a single session, three times a day (morning, noon, and evening). The pressure should be moderate. A treatment course consists of 6 months. A combination of Chinese and Western medicine treatment plans has shown good therapeutic effects.

Epilepsy is a common and prevalent disease that has imposed a heavy burden on society, families, and patients. The treatment of epilepsy has attracted widespread attention, leading to significant advancements in its management. TCM has its unique advantages in treating epilepsy and plays an irreplaceable role in its treatment. TCM itself has experienced rapid development, particularly in recent years with the emergence of new treatment theories and methods. The continuous progress in modern scientific level has driven improvements in medical facilities and substantial advancements in medical practices, resulting in diverse treatment methods and significant outcomes. The application of various treatment methods in clinical practice has brought about gratifying achievements for patients, especially in the realm of TCM treatment. In the future, continuous exploration and research are needed in the clinical diagnosis and treatment of epilepsy to help more epilepsy patients.

2.3 Practice of Epilepsy Management in Women with Epilepsy of Childbearing Age

Yutong Fu

2.3.1 Challenges and Practices in Epilepsy Management for Women of Childbearing Age

The prevalence of WWE in China is estimated to be 3.45 per 1000 population, ranging from 2.83 to 3.14 per 1000 women of childbearing age (defined as age 20–40 years). WWE of childbearing age face multifaceted challenges throughout various stages of their life cycle, requiring comprehensive interdisciplinary management. During adolescence, hormonal changes may trigger reproductive dysfunction such as polycystic ovary syndrome (PCOS), infertility, or affect neuronal excitability and cause catamenial epilepsy. Effective contraception for women of childbearing potential is important as many antiseizure medications (ASMs) affect the unborn fetus and interact with steroid hormones. However, women requiring contraception may encounter limitations in contraceptive selection or effectiveness due to interactions between ASMs and contraceptives as well as the association between contraceptives and seizure deterioration. During the preconception phase, optimal seizure control, appropriate folate supplementation, and adjustments of ASM regimens are imperative. Profound physiological changes that occur during pregnancy lead to fluctuations in ASM concentrations and increased risks of seizures and status epilepticus, threatening both maternal and fetal health. Additionally, ASM intake during pregnancy is associated with adverse outcomes including congenital malformations, birth defects, and neurodevelopmental delays. For decisions regarding the childbirth delivery mode, the impact of labor pain stimulation or anesthesia on epilepsy management must be considered. The postpartum period also presents challenges relating to breastfeeding decisions, outbreak of emotional disorders like depression, and long-term developmental concerns for offspring. Therefore, multidisciplinary collaboration involving specialists in neurology, gynecology, obstetrics, pediatrics, genetics, anesthesiology, pharmacy, and other relevant fields is paramount for addressing the challenges and offering effective interventions to support WWE across their entire lifespan.

Our team has spearheaded the holistic management of WWE of childbearing age, as illustrated in Fig. 2.3. Through a chronic disease management system, we have streamlined the rapid retrieval and export of patient records. Furthermore, our patients benefit from the expertise of specialized physicians who guide them through the entire management process, facilitating better communication between healthcare providers and patients. Additionally, we prioritize disease-specific and targeted education for patients to enhance their understanding and engagement. Over the past decade, our efforts have led to significant clinical improvements, including a

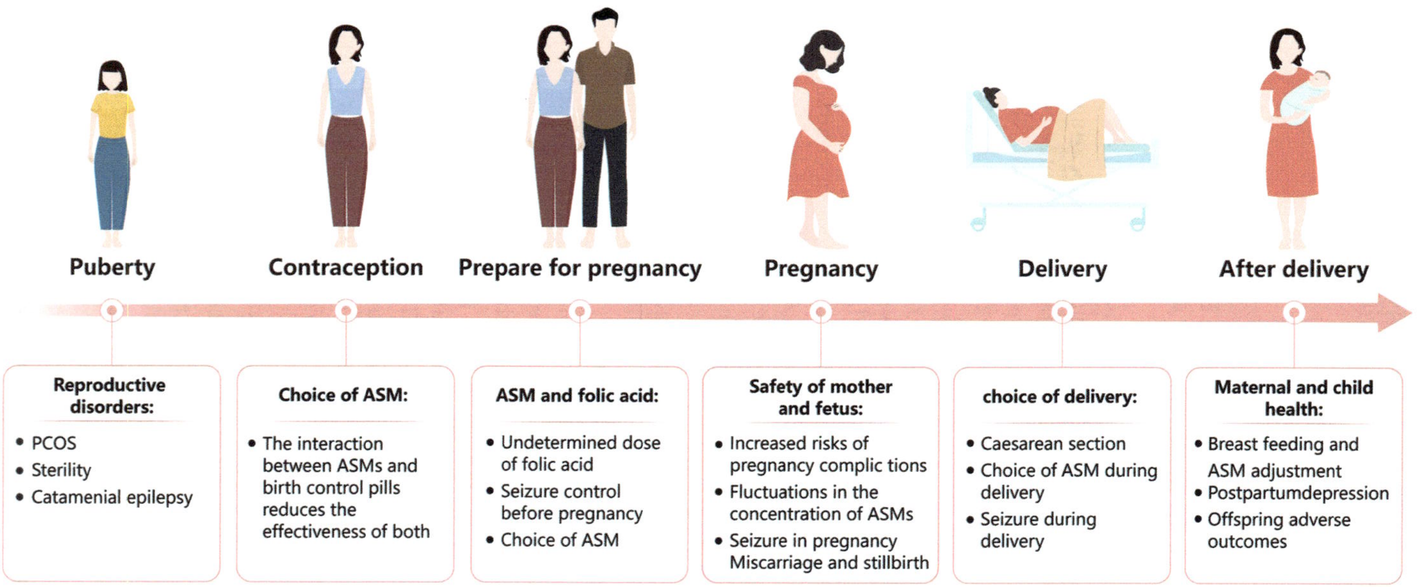

Fig. 2.3 Challenges throughout various stages of their life in women with epilepsy of childbearing age

relatively 17.2% reduction in infertility rates, a relatively 0.04% decrease in pregnancy-related mortality, a relatively 6.4% decrease in the incidence of congenital malformations, and a relatively 1% reduction in stillbirth rates.

Furthermore, given the chronic nature of epilepsy and the challenges associated with long-term adherence to ASM regimens, prioritizing patient- and family-centered care is essential. Our team has implemented a variety of educational initiatives aimed to improve the adherence of patients and their families. First, we wrote Chinese first popular science book on epilepsy in women of childbearing age, providing guidance and advice on scientific planning for pregnancy, pregnancy management, safe delivery, and proper child-rearing practices. With rich illustrations, this chapter seeks to improve patients' understanding of the disease and instill their confidence in achieving healthy pregnancies. Second, we pioneered live broadcasts of support groups for WWE of childbearing age. These sessions invite peer experts and reproductive endocrinologists to educate patients and their families on the possibility and information on safe and healthy pregnancy. Third, we offered free clinical services offline to provide face-to-face educational opportunities to patients, especially in remote regions such as Aba and Ganzi in Sichuan Province, as well as in western regions such as Tibet, Yunnan, and Guizhou. Additionally, our team produces educational microfilms and has used various social media platforms for dissemination. For instance, our microfilm "Lights" told the story of a girl with epilepsy who grew up to become a mother, inspiring WWE to bravely embrace motherhood. This microfilm has garnered over 70,000 views on the Weibo video channel of West China Hospital, Sichuan University. In the digital age, we also harness the benefits of digital technologies to deliver multidimensional education and raise awareness of self-health management. For instance, we deliver message reminders to improve ASM adherence. Patients are required to complete electronic diaries to document their seizures and ASM use, which helps them to develop good habits. On the other hand, the intelligent assistants in the system can help address patients' queries and bridge knowledge gaps. Physicians can also access real-time patient data for making well-informed decisions during following consultations. Through these initiatives, our team aims to empower WWE and their families with the knowledge and tools necessary for effective epilepsy management and improved quality of life.

To effectively support women of childbearing age facing the challenges of epilepsy, our team has established the first multidisciplinary clinic for WWE in China. This platform aims to address various concerns specific to women of childbearing age, including reproductive endocrine issues, comorbid mental health disorders, genetic considerations, pregnancy-related difficulties, childbirth consultations, infant feeding methods, and neurodevelopmental aspects. Patients from multiple centers, multidisciplinary clinics, and community populations across the country can benefit from this remote consultation platform, which provides comprehensive, individualized, and precise diagnosis and treatment services. Through this whole-course approach, we aim to provide continuous health management services for women of childbearing age with epilepsy, ensuring their overall well-being and quality of life.

2.3.2 Explorations of Novel Mechanisms of Drug-Resistant Epilepsy from Extracerebral Systems

Drug-resistant epilepsy is the most common reason of uncontrolled seizures and polytherapy for pregnant women with epilepsy, which bring great burden for both mothers with epilepsy and their offspring. Our team have been working to explore mechanisms of refractory epilepsy from extracerebral systems through brain-peripheral organs interactions.

2.3.2.1 Relationship Between Patent Foramen Ovale (PFO) and Epilepsy

Patent foramen ovale (PFO) is a common congenital heart defect characterized by an incomplete closure of the septum primum and secundum. PFO facilitates right-to-left shunting of blood, allowing for unoxygenated venous blood and micro-emboli passage from the venous to the arterial circulation, potentially leading to hypoxemia. PFO can also cause cerebral endothelial dysfunction, cortical excitability changes, and ischemic or hypoxic insults, increasing susceptibility to stroke, migraine, and obstructive sleep apnea. Previous studies have found that chronic hypoxia leads to elevated neuronal excitability, which may decrease seizure threshold and contribute to refractory epilepsy, with seizure-associated hypoxemia also being a potential mechanism for SUDEP. Among patients with seizures of unclear origin referred to our epilepsy clinic by cardiologists, we have encountered a number of patients with prominent PFO who were ultimately diagnosed as having epilepsy. In addition, we have observed that the frequency of seizures seems to significantly reduce in some patients after PFO closure.

To further validate our hypothesis, our team conducted contrast transesophageal echocardiography (cTTE) in 604 patients with epilepsy (PWE), revealing a right left shunt (RLS) prevalence of up to 47.2% among patients with refractory epilepsy (Dong et al. 2023a; Tang et al. 2023). After accounting for other risk factors associated with refractory epilepsy, RLS remained a potentially independent risk factor. Additionally, refractory epilepsy patients with RLS demonstrated lower arterial oxygen partial pressure compared to those without RLS, suggesting a potential underlying mechanism for refractory epilepsy. Our team further conducted a comparative analysis between PWE and a control group without epilepsy and found the risk of PFO in PWE to be 1.71 times higher than in controls, with an increased risk of obtaining higher RLS grades. Additionally, PWE with PFO were more likely to be diagnosed with RE as well as comorbid migraine. Based on these findings, we proposed a novel hypothesis to explore the efficacy of PFO closure surgery in treating refractory epilepsy. Among 16 PWE who underwent PFO closure surgery, nine cases (56.3%) experienced a reduction in seizure frequency postoperatively. Importantly, three patients with refractory epilepsy showed symptom improvement without ASM adjustments. While further large-scale multicenter studies are required to validate these findings, our team has provided new insights into the potential association between PFO and epilepsy, which may have implications for the management of PWE.

To investigate the potential mechanisms through which PFO affects epilepsy, we collected plasma samples from the peripheral blood of PWE before and 1 year after surgery, as well as blood samples from the right and left atria collected during surgery, for proteomic analysis. Protein profiling studies reveal elevated levels of hemoglobin and cell adhesion molecules in right atrial blood after PFO closure, indicating improved oxygen transport. Additionally, in vitro experiments have demonstrated increased levels of oxidative stress-related proteins in the occipital lobe of PFO-positive mice, suggesting a role of PFO-induced intermittent hypoxia in oxidative stress development (Dong et al. 2023b).

Therefore, integrating multi-site and timepoint proteomics with clinical outcomes and mice model data supports the hypothesis that PFO closure surgery prevents RLS and alleviates hypoxia, potentially restoring protein homeostasis in the brain and benefiting epilepsy patients.

2.3.2.2 Relationship Between Polycystic Ovary Syndrome (PCOS) and Epilepsy

The management of WWE presents distinctive challenges owing to the intricate interactions between women's hormonal secretions, seizure control, and the metabolism of ASMs. On the one hand, the influence of female steroid hormone on neuronal excitability can render individuals more susceptible to triggered epileptic seizures associated with hormonal cycles. On the other hand, both seizures and ASMs can interfere with ovarian function, impair hormone secretion, and adversely affect the reproductive health of WWE, resulting in higher infertility and reproductive dysfunction. PCOS is a prevalent disorder among women of reproductive age, recognized as a leading cause of anovulatory infertility. PCOS has emerged as a significant comorbidity in epilepsy, with studies reporting a higher prevalence (15–30%) among WWE compared to the general female population (5–20%). The co-occurrence of PCOS in WWE is associated with metabolic abnormalities such as dyslipidemia, hyperglycemia, and insulin resistance, which can increase the risk of long-term complications including obesity, diabetes, and cardiovascular disease. Therefore, the early identification of PCOS and personalized management strategies are crucial for optimizing reproductive health and mitigating metabolic risks in WWE.

To explore the clinical risk factors and characteristics for WWE with PCOS, our team screened 238 WWE with PCOS, providing a comprehensive analysis of PCOS risk factors in women with epilepsy, focusing on medical history, ASM intake, and hormone levels (Lai et al. 2023). Our results revealed that prolonged use of levetiracetam for over 1 year, obesity, high luteinizing hormone, and anti-Müllerian hormone levels were independent risk factors for comorbid PCOS. Additionally, characteristic features of WWE with PCOS included epilepsy onset before age 13, perinatal asphyxia, low sex hormone-binding globulin levels, and elevated cholesterol levels. Our findings indicated that WWE with comorbid PCOS experienced higher seizure frequency compared to those without PCOS, potentially attributable to the impact of PCOS on brain function and increased risk of refractory epilepsy. Based on our findings, we introduced the "Early Prevention, Early Detection, and Early Treatment" protocol for WWE with comorbid PCOS. This protocol emphasizes the importance of early screening for PCOS during adolescence, as well as the cautious avoidance of ASMs that impact the gonadal axis in children. Additionally, prompt initiation of PCOS treatment is advocated. Standardized PCOS management, inclusive of hormone therapy, is recommended as it not only enhances fertility but also contributes to mitigating the severity of epilepsy.

Innovatively, our team conducted functional magnetic resonance imaging (fMRI) scans on newly diagnosed, untreated PCOS patients, revealing reduced functional connectivity in the right frontal lobe associated with elevated luteinizing hormone levels. This finding implies that PCOS may induce alterations in brain activity and connectivity in regions responsible for visual-spatial working memory, facial processing, and episodic memory. From genetic insights, our team identified shared susceptibility genes in WWE comorbid with PCOS through whole-genome sequencing, including ZFTVE28, SIK3, COL19A1, PPIG, ANKK1, and REPIN1. Notably, ZFTVE28 and PPIG were implicated for the first time in both epilepsy and PCOS. Additionally, we observed a significant enrichment of susceptibility genes related to insulin metabolism pathways in epileptic women with PCOS, highlighting the crucial role of insulin metabolism dysfunction in the development of epilepsy comorbid with PCOS. Therefore, we proposed that early genetic screening of WWE may help identify individuals who are more likely to develop PCOS and allow for prompt risk-reduction interventions.

2.3.2.3 Relationship Between Gastrointestinal Function and Epilepsy

The bidirectional regulation of the gut–brain axis has emerged as a research hotspot in recent years. The central nervous system (CNS) regulates gastrointestinal function through sympathetic and parasympathetic pathways. Conversely, the gastrointestinal tract can also influence the CNS through various mechanisms, including the vagal reflex and metabolites from the gut microbiota. Traditional medicine in China has long proposed the theory of "disorder of the stomach leading to insomnia with restlessness" and "if the stomach is dry and the stool is hard, one is delirious," recognizing the connection between gastrointestinal health and CNS disorders. Similarly, Western medicine also has described the concept of the gut–brain axis, all of which highlight the importance of maintaining gut homeostasis for overall well-being. Emerging research indicates that gastrointestinal dysfunction can contribute to the development of CNS disorders, including autism, Parkinson's disease, and schizophrenia.

Our team previously analyzed microbiome composition through high-throughput sequencing of bacterial 16s ribosomal DNA (rDNA) (Peng et al. 2018). We observed that dysbiosis may be implicated in the pathogenesis of refractory epilepsy, with notably increased abundance of rare bacterial taxa such as *Clostridium difficile* in the gut microbiota of patients with refractory epilepsy (Nucera et al. 2022). Consequently, we proposed that restoring gut microbiota homeostasis may represent a potential therapeutic approach for treating refractory epilepsy, and further developed a protocol involving the appropriate ratio of probiotics and prebiotics as a treatment strategy for refractory epilepsy.

Furthermore, we have performed electrogastrography (EGG), a non-invasive technique, to record gastrointestinal myoelectrical activity. EGG has been used as an auxiliary diagnostic tool for various functional gastrointestinal disorders, offering an accurate and objective assessment of gastrointestinal function in participants. Our previous research identified gastric dysrhythmia in patients with cognitive dysfunction and sleep disorders. Based on gastric electrical parameters, we successfully developed predictive statistical models for these above-mentioned diseases, and demonstrated its robust and stable predictive performance. These achievements provide additional evidence to support the brain–gut axis theory. Currently, we are exploring the specific gastrointestinal electrophysiologic signals in patients with refractory epilepsy, and attempting to integrate traditional Chinese medical techniques to explore the potential of performing acupuncture at certain abdominal acupoints to alleviate seizure frequency.

2.3.3 Innovative Strategies for ASM Management During Pregnancy

Most women with epilepsy continue ASM treatments during pregnancy. Our team have been working to provide more effective ASM management during pregnancy for Chinese women with epilepsy.

2.3.3.1 Risk Assessments of ASM Use in Pregnancy

The use of ASMs during pregnancy is associated with specific risks to the fetus, and teratogenicity is one of the main concerns. Assessing the teratogenic risks of ASMs is crucial in ensuring the safety of pregnant individuals and their offspring. Using US Food and Drug Administration (FDA)-approved drug labels, our team identified a list of ASMs with potential teratogenic risks and constructed a support vector machine (SVM) model to detect drugs with high teratogenicity. Validation of the model was conducted using post-market surveillance data from the US FDA Spontaneous Adverse Events Reporting System (FAERS). Our analysis identified four commonly used ASMs with high predicted teratogenic risks, including topiramate, phenobarbital, valproate, and phenytoin, aligning with existing FDA label and pregnancy and epilepsy registry reports. Additionally, newer ASMs such as perampanel, lacosamide, and brivaracetam were also predicted to have high risks. The model demonstrated robust performance in predicting teratogenic risks and facilitated the evaluation of potential teratogenic risks for newly approved ASMs, providing valuable insights to support clinical decision-making. By accurately identifying drugs with high teratogenicity, this approach supports precision medicine in relation to ASM customization and contributes to safer medication practices during pregnancy.

Additionally, our team found that optimal co-administration of ASMs and folic acid reduced offspring malformations. Folic acid supplementation during pregnancy is widely recommended to prevent the risk of various adverse pregnancy outcomes, including low birth weight, preterm birth, miscarriage, and preeclampsia. Notably, folic acid deficiency has been associated with an increased risk of neural tube defects in offspring. However, the simultaneous use of folic acid with certain ASMs may present challenges due to potential interactions affecting both folate metabolism and ASM efficacy. The long-term use of ASMs, particularly enzyme-inducing ASMs, may affect serum folate metabolism and potentially lead to folic acid deficiency during pregnancy. Conversely, studies have also suggested that folic acid supplementation may diminish the efficacy of lamotrigine, a commonly prescribed ASM. Our analysis has revealed striking similarities in the amino acid residue positions and spatial orientations where lamotrigine binds to the transporter compared to folic acid, indicating a competitive relationship. Novel ASMs should prioritize reducing interactions with folic acid to reduce dosage requirements, and enhance blood–brain barrier targeting to reduce placental permeability, thereby minimizing fetal exposure and potential adverse effects.

2.3.3.2 Monitoring of ASM Concentrations in Pregnancy

Pregnancy induces physiological changes in the maternal body, leading to potential alterations in the dose–response relationship of ASMs. Consequently, the originally prescribed doses may become ineffective or result in new adverse outcomes. Given the impact of fluctuations in ASM concentrations on fetal exposure and maternal seizure control, understanding the changes in pharmacokinetics of ASMs during pregnancy is crucial. Physiology-based pharmacokinetics (PBPK) modeling is characterized by its mechanistic and physiology-driven approach, and is often employed in early drug development to predict a drug's behavior, simulate dosing regimens, and guide dosage and formulation decisions. It holds significant value in predicting pharmacokinetics and ASM exposure in both mother and fetus during pregnancy. Our team has constructed nonlinear mixed-effects models for different ASMs using blood and saliva concentrations collected before, during, and after pregnancy. By incorporating these data into PBPK models, we developed pregnancy-specific clearance-concentration standard curves for different ASMs. These models enable dose simulations tailored to individual patient characteristics and clinical scenarios, optimizing drug regimens during pregnancy.

Traditional methods of measuring ASM concentrations in plasma or serum remain the preferred approach for therapeutic drug monitoring. However, frequent blood sampling can cause patients physical discomfort and reduce their compliance.

Our team has made an effort to explore simpler, non-invasive, and reproducible alternative sources, and achieved measurements through the use of saliva. Previous research has demonstrated positive correlations between saliva and plasma concentrations for commonly used ASMs in WWE during pregnancy, including levetiracetam, lamotrigine, and oxcarbazepine metabolites. Therefore, saliva can serve as an effective alternative for blood in monitoring ASM concentrations in pregnant women with epilepsy. In addition to innovative detection techniques, we have also developed novel detection devices through nanopore sensor technology, enabling point-of-care testing (POCT) for real-time monitoring of medication concentrations and at-home testing. Traditional processes for measuring ASM concentrations are complex, involving large and costly instrumentation, which is unsuitable for pregnant WWE and the implementation of drug concentration monitoring in primary healthcare settings. Therefore, our team has designed nanopore sensing devices, based on the molecular characteristics of ASMs and the structural features of their targets within the body. Integrated with microfluidic technology, these devices enable the continuous monitoring of ASM concentrations and facilitate the testing of various body fluid samples. Furthermore, POCT technology offers advantages such as small size, high-throughput, real-time sensing, and low costs, simplifying the testing process and achieving convenient, at-home monitoring of drug concentrations with rapid results.

2.3.4 Innovative Technologies for Epilepsy Monitoring and Prediction

Uncontrolled seizure during pregnancy could be associated with lethal incidents of both mothers with epilepsy and their fetus. Effective monitoring and prediction of seizure during pregnancy could improve life quality of pregnant women with epilepsy. Our team have been working to establish a more effective system for epilepsy monitoring and prediction.

2.3.4.1 Establishment of a Remote Seizure Monitoring and Alert System

Epileptic seizures are often sudden and abrupt, and can be accompanied by a loss of consciousness in patients. Witnesses are often startled and unable to accurately describe details or record the event, which may impact the diagnosis and treatment of epilepsy. Moreover, seizures can lead to injuries, particularly in pregnant WWE, posing risks to both the mother and fetus. Therefore, the development of a system capable of remotely detecting seizures and sending real-time alerts to family members or caregivers could potentially reduce the harms caused by seizures.

To address this issue, our team has developed a remote monitoring and alert system based on behavioral recognition technology to detect epileptic seizures in real-time and provide timely interventions. The system uses artificial intelligence (AI) algorithms to analyze video footage captured by smart cameras installed throughout the home. By detecting abnormal motion trajectories associated with epileptic seizures, the AI can accurately identify seizure events. Subsequently, the system analyzes the video, anonymizes the images, and sends alerts to the designated contacts for prompt intervention, thereby preventing further harm. This behavioral recognition technology enables the system to distinguish epileptic seizures from other movements or activities, ensuring reliable detection and minimizing false alarms. This intelligent alert system can be widely applied not only in hospitals but also in homes and communities, offering people a safer and more convenient living environment.

2.3.4.2 Development of Seizure Warning Urine Protein and Metabolomics Kits

Urinary biomarkers offer several advantages for clinical diagnostics and disease monitoring. First, urine collection is convenient and easily accessible, making it a practical and non-invasive sampling method. Second, urine composition is not subject to the regulatory mechanisms that govern blood composition, making it a more stable matrix for biomarker analysis. Furthermore, urinary proteins and metabolites have been identified as potential biomarkers for various neurological disorders, such as stroke, brain tumors, Alzheimer's disease, and Parkinson's disease, offering the possibility of early detection and intervention.

Our team have proposed a novel approach using urinary proteomic and metabolomic analysis to identify distinct alterations that predict seizures, offering a non-invasive and potentially more accurate method for seizure prediction. We conducted tests in patients with refractory epilepsy, collecting morning urine samples on a daily basis and additional samples obtained postictally.

2.3.4.3 Establishment of an Out-of-Hospital Smart Visualized System for Epilepsy Emergency Follow-Up and Treatment

The development of novel technologies for epileptic seizure prediction represents a significant advancement in epilepsy management. In addition to technology and systems used for seizure prediction, our team has also constructed an out-of-hospital smart visualization system for epilepsy emergency follow-up and treatment. Patients with seizures lasting more than 4 min or experiencing other emergency situations are promptly transferred to the hospital for a more comprehensive assessment and specialized emergency measures. The entire process is illustrated in Fig. 2.4.

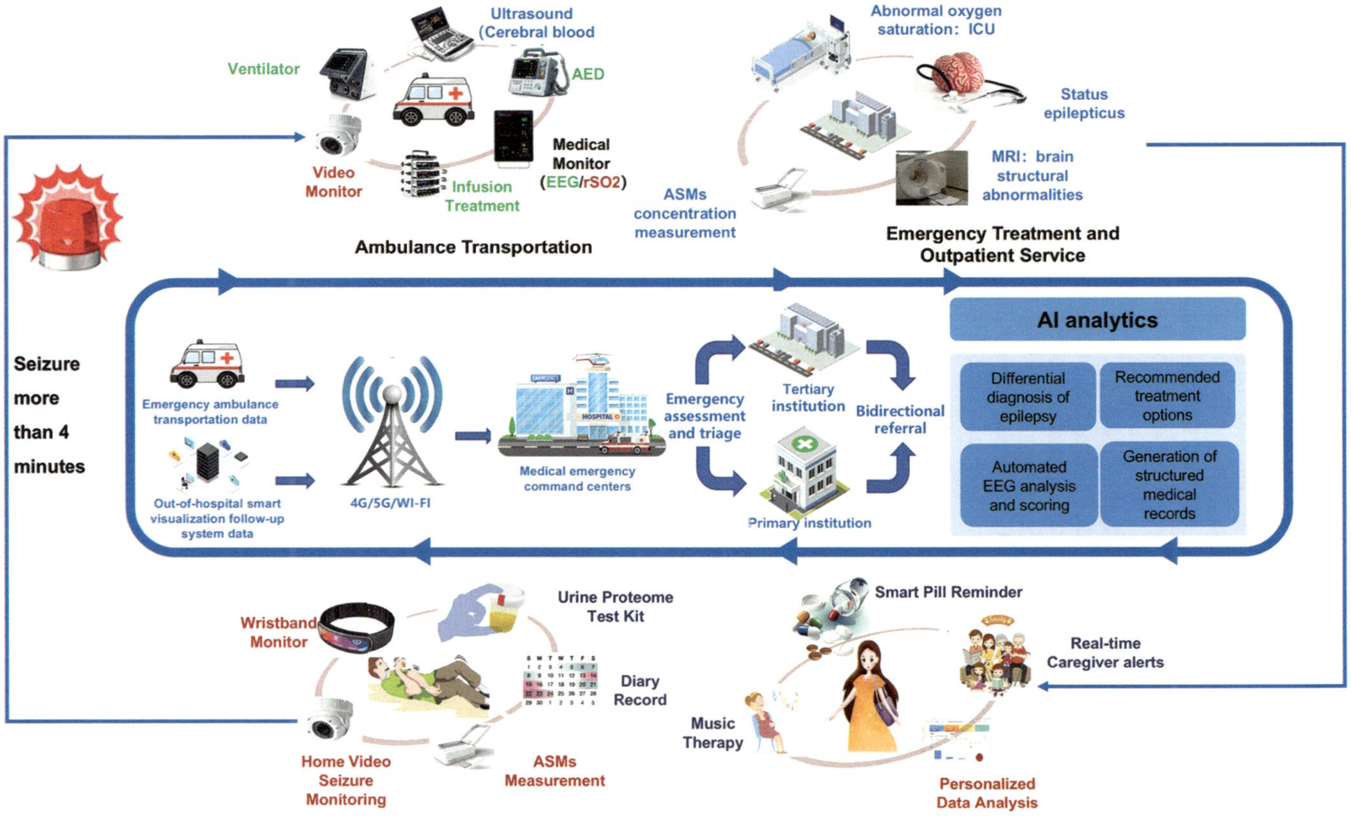

Fig. 2.4 The whole process of out-of-hospital smart visualization for epilepsy emergency treatment. *AED* automated external defibrillator, *EEG* electroencephalogram, rSO_2 regional oxygen saturation, *ICU* intensive care units, *ASM* antiseizure medication, *AI* artificial intelligence, *MRI* magnetic resonance imaging

References

Dong B, Li Y, Ji S, He S, Lai Q, Yang X, et al. Relationship between right-to-left shunt, hypoxia, and epilepsy. Epilepsia Open. 2023a;8:456–65.

Dong B, Lu Y, He S, Li B, Li Y, Lai Q, et al. Multisite and multitimepoint proteomics reveal that patent foramen ovale closure improves migraine and epilepsy by reducing right-to-left shunt-induced hypoxia. MedComm. 2023b;4:e334.

Lai W, Shen N, Zhu H, He S, Yang X, Lai Q, et al. Identifying risk factors for polycystic ovary syndrome in women with epilepsy: a comprehensive analysis of 248 patients. J Neuroendocrinol. 2023;35:e13250.

Nucera B, Brigo F, Trinka E, Kalss G. Treatment and care of women with epilepsy before, during, and after pregnancy: a practical guide. Ther Adv Neurol Disord. 2022;15:17562864221101687.

Peng A, Qiu X, Lai W, Li W, Zhang L, Zhu X, et al. Altered composition of the gut microbiome in patients with drug-resistant epilepsy. Epilepsy Res. 2018;147:102–7.

Tang Y, Ji S, Li H, Dong B, Li Y, Zhu C, et al. Association of patent foramen ovale with epilepsy: a hospital-based case–control study. Epilepsia Open. 2023;8:1075–83.

Suggested Readings

Alvestad S, Husebye ESN, Christensen J, Dreier JW, Sun Y, Igland J, et al. Folic acid and risk of preterm birth, preeclampsia, and fetal growth restriction among women with epilepsy. Neurology. 2022;99:e605–15.

Amini L, Hematian M, Montazeri A, Gharegozli K. Comparing the frequency of polycystic ovary syndrome in women with and without epilepsy. J Family Med Prim Care. 2018;7:16–20.

An M, Gao Y. Urinary biomarkers of brain diseases. Genomics Proteomics Bioinformatics. 2015;13:345–54.

Avram MJ. Pharmacokinetic studies in pregnancy. Semin Perinatol. 2020;44:151227.

Balen AH, Morley LC, Misso M, Franks S, Legro RS, Wijeyaratne CN, et al. The management of anovulatory infertility in women with polycystic ovary syndrome: an analysis of the evidence to support the development of global WHO guidance. Hum Reprod Update. 2016;22:687–708.

Bilo L, Meo R, Valentino R, Carlo CD, Striano S, Nappi C. Characterization of reproductive endocrine disorders in women with epilepsy. J Clin Endocrinol Metab. 2001;86:2950.

Buchanan GF, Maciel ATN, Summerfield M. Sudden unexpected death in epilepsy. Curr Opin Neurol. 2022;35:181–8.

Charlson FJ, Baxter AJ, Cheng HG, Shidhaye R, Whiteford HA. The burden of mental, neurological, and substance use disorders in China and India: a systematic analysis of community representative epidemiological studies. Lancet. 2016;388:376–89.

Cryan JF, O'Riordan KJ, Cowan CSM, Sandhu KV, Bastiaanssen TFS, Boehme M, et al. The microbiota-gut-brain axis. Physiol Rev. 2019;99:1877–2013.

Devinsky O, Vezzani A, O'Brien TJ, Jette N, Scheffer IE, de Curtis M, et al. Epilepsy. Nat Rev Dis Primers. 2018;4:18024.

Ding D, Zhou D, Sander JW, Wang W, Li S, Hong Z. Epilepsy in China: major progress in the past two decades. Lancet Neurol. 2021;20:316–26.

Geddes JR, Gardiner A, Rendell J, Voysey M, Tunbridge E, Hinds C, et al. Comparative evaluation of quetiapine plus lamotrigine combination versus quetiapine monotherapy (and folic acid versus placebo) in bipolar depression (CEQUEL): a 2 × 2 factorial randomised trial. Lancet Psychiatry. 2016;3:31–9.

Generoso JS, Giridharan VV, Lee J, Macedo D, Barichello T. The role of the microbiota-gut-brain axis in neuropsychiatric disorders. Braz J Psychiatry. 2020;43:293–305.

Giblett JP, Williams LK, Kyranis S, Shapiro LM, Calvert PA. Patent foramen ovale closure: state of the art. Interv Cardiol. 2020;15:e15.

Gu L, Liang B, Chen Q, Long L, Xie L, Wu G, et al. Prevalence of epilepsy in the People's Republic of China: a systematic review. Epilepsy Res. 2013;105:195–205.

Ji S, Li B, Zhu C, Jiang G, Tang Y, Chen L. Risk assessment model for sleep disturbance based on gastrointestinal myoelectrical activity in middle-aged and elderly people. Front Psych. 2023;14:1183108.

Joshi S, Kapur J. Neurosteroid regulation of GABAA receptors: a role in catamenial epilepsy. Brain Res. 2019;1703:31–40.

Kang L, Duan Y, Chen C, Li S, Li M, Chen L, et al. Structure-activity relationship (SAR) model for predicting teratogenic risk of antiseizure medications in pregnancy by using support vector machine. Front Pharmacol. 2022;13:747935.

Karaś-Ruszczyk K, Kuczyńska J, Sienkiewicz-Jarosz H, Kurkowska-Jastrzębska I, Bienkowski P, Restel M, et al. Comparison of plasma, saliva, and hair levetiracetam concentrations. Ther Drug Monit. 2017;39:263–8.

Kuczynska J, Karas-Ruszczyk K, Zakrzewska A, Dermanowski M, Sienkiewicz-Jarosz H, Kurkowska-Jastrzebska I, et al. Comparison of plasma, saliva, and hair lamotrigine concentrations. Clin Biochem. 2019;74:24–30.

Kutty S, Sengupta PP, Khandheria BK. Patent foramen ovale: the known and the to be known. J Am Coll Cardiol. 2012;59:1665–71.

Lai W, Li X, Zhu H, Zhu X, Tan H, Feng P, et al. Plasma luteinizing hormone level affects the brain activity of patients with polycystic ovary syndrome. Psychoneuroendocrinology. 2020;112:104535.

Levin-Epstein R, Kumar P, Rusheen J, Fleming RG, McWatters Z, Kim W, et al. Investigation of patent foramen ovale as a mechanism for brain metastasis in patients without prior lung involvement. Clin Transl Oncol. 2021;23:783–7.

Li B, Ji S, Peng A, Yang N, Zhao X, Feng P, et al. Development of a gastrointestinal-myoelectrical-activity-based nomogram model for predicting the risk of mild cognitive impairment. Biomolecules. 2022;12:1861.

Linnebank M, Moskau S, Semmler A, Widman G, Stoffel-Wagner B, Weller M, et al. Antiepileptic drugs interact with folate and vitamin B12 serum levels. Ann Neurol. 2011;69:352–9.

Liu J, Wu Q, Hao Y, Jiao M, Wang X, Jiang S, et al. Measuring the global disease burden of polycystic ovary syndrome in 194 countries: Global Burden of Disease Study 2017. Hum Reprod. 2021;36:1108–19.

Luef G, Abraham I, Haslinger M, Trinka E, Seppi K, Unterberger I, et al. Polycystic ovaries, obesity and insulin resistance in women with epilepsy. J Neurol. 2002;249:835–41.

Morais LH, Schreiber HL, Mazmanian SK. The gut microbiota–brain axis in behaviour and brain disorders. Nat Rev Microbiol. 2021;19:241–55.

Patsalos PN, Berry DJ. Therapeutic drug monitoring of antiepileptic drugs by use of saliva. Ther Drug Monit. 2013;35:4.

Peigné M, Dewailly D. Long term complications of polycystic ovary syndrome (PCOS). Ann Endocrinol. 2014;75:194–9.

Peng A, Wang R, Huang J, Wu H, Chen L. Abnormalities of resting-state electroencephalographic microstate in rapid eye movement sleep behavior disorder. Front Hum Neurosci. 2021;15:728405.

Socała K, Doboszewska U, Szopa A, Serefko A, Włodarczyk M, Zielińska A, et al. The role of microbiota-gut-brain axis in neuropsychiatric and neurological disorders. Pharmacol Res. 2021;172:105840.

Tomson T, Battino D, Bonizzoni E, Craig J, Lindhout D, Perucca E, et al. Comparative risk of major congenital malformations with eight different antiepileptic drugs: a prospective cohort study of the EURAP registry. Lancet Neurol. 2018;17:530–8.

WHO. Epilepsy: a public health imperative. Geneva: World Health Organization; 2019.

Xu Y, Fan Q. Relationship between chronic hypoxia and seizure susceptibility. CNS Neurosci Ther. 2022;28:1689–705.

Yang R, Li Q, Zhou Z, Qian W, Zhang J, Wu Z, et al. Changes in the prevalence of polycystic ovary syndrome in China over the past decade. Lancet Reg Health West Pac. 2022;25:100494.

Yin J, Chen JDZ. Electrogastrography: methodology, validation and applications. J Neurogastroenterol Motil. 2013;19:5–17.

Zhou J-Q, Zhou L-M, Chen L-J, Han J-D, Wang Q, Fang Z-Y, et al. Polycystic ovary syndrome in patients with epilepsy: a study in 102 Chinese women. Seizure. 2012;21:729–33.

The Relationship Between Epilepsy, Antiseizure Medication, and Sex Hormones

3

Ziyi Chen and Leihao Sha

3.1 Seizures and Sex Hormones

Ziyi Chen and Leihao Sha

The results of animal experiments show that epileptic seizures can cause increased estrogen levels, but clinical observational studies show that the level of blood E2 and free E2 in female epileptic patients is significantly lower than that in normal women, regardless of whether they are in the follicular phase or luteal phase of the menstrual cycle. In terms of seizure type, most studies have focused on patients with focal epilepsy and temporal lobe epilepsy (TLE), finding that E2 levels were significantly lower than that of control groups, and the E2 level in patients with right-sided TLE was lower than that in patients with left-sided TLE. In terms of seizure frequency, the level of free E2 during the luteal phase in patients with high seizure frequency was significantly lower than that in normal women. In both follicular and luteal phases, P levels in the blood of epilepsy patients were significantly lower than normal controls, and P levels in the luteal phase of patients with high seizure frequency were significantly lower than that in normal women. Meletti et al. also found that P levels in the cerebrospinal fluid of patients with status epilepticus were significantly lower than normal controls. The most studied androgens in WWE include T, DHEAS, and androstenedione. In terms of epilepsy type, levels of DHEAS have been found to be significantly higher in female patients with TLE than in normal controls. From the point of view of seizure frequency, patients with higher seizure

Z. Chen (✉)
Department of Neurology, The First Affiliated Hospital, Sun Yat-sen University, Guangzhou, China
e-mail: chenziyi@mail.sysu.edu.cn

L. Sha
Department of Neurology, West China Hospital, Sichuan University, Chengdu, China

L. Chen (ed.), *Women with Epilepsy in Child-bearing Age*,
https://doi.org/10.1007/978-981-97-3921-9_3

frequency have been associated with lower DHEAS levels, while from the point of view of lesion location, T levels in patients with right-sided TLE have been shown to be significantly lower than those in controls and patients with left-sided TLE. Studies evaluating the effect of epilepsy on prolactin (PRL) levels have focused on the elevation of PRL in the short period following seizures. In 1976, Ohman et al. reported that serum PRL levels increased 10–50-fold in 8 out of 9 depressed patients 15 min after electroconvulsive therapy. In 1978, Trimble described elevated PRL levels in patients with epilepsy after surgery. Subsequently, researchers have shown that serum PRL levels may rise briefly after systemic motor and partial seizures, peaking within 15–20 min and gradually returning to baseline levels within the next hour. The incidence of elevated PRL levels after seizures has been associated with seizure type. Using deep electrodes and video monitoring, Sperling et al. found that PRL levels increased more than two-fold after seizures that resulted in widespread high-frequency electrical activity in the medial temporal limbic region, but not after seizures that did not involve limbic structures that trigger PRL release. In contrast, Wyllie et al. and Bauer et al. found that serum PRL levels were elevated after 80% of total tonic-clonic seizures, 39–43% of complex partial seizures, and only 10% of simple partial seizures. In addition, PRL levels were not elevated in patients with absence seizures or status epilepticus. The study found that the average basal FSH level in WWE was significantly higher than that in the normal control group, while the pulse frequency of LH was significantly elevated in WWE, resulting in a shortened interval between the LH pulses, so seizures may interfere with GnRH pulse occurrence activity. In terms of seizure type, elevated levels of LH and FSH in the blood were detected 20 min after a general seizure in female patients and remained elevated 60 min after the seizure but were not observed in patients with complex partial seizures. The ratio of LH/FSH was higher in patients with idiopathic generalized epilepsy (IGE) than in patients with focal-related epilepsy (LGE) than in normal controls. From the focal epilepsy perspective, the LH/FSH ratio in patients with left TLE has been identified as significantly higher than that in patients with right TLE, because the FSH levels in patients with left TLE were lower than those in patients with right TLE.

3.2 Antiseizure Medications and Sex Hormones

Ziyi Chen and Leihao Sha

In addition to the epileptic disease itself having an impact on female sex hormones, ASMs can also exacerbate reproductive endocrine dysfunction in women with epilepsy. ASMs can directly inhibit reproductive function by regulating the release of sex hormones through the hypothalamic-pituitary-gonadal axis, and the ASMs can also alter the metabolism of sex hormones and their binding proteins.

Studies have shown that enzyme-inducing antiepileptic drugs such as carbamazepine, phenytoin, phenobarbital, and oxcarbazepine can promote the synthesis of sex hormone-binding proteins, promote the metabolism of androgens, and produce a large amount of estrogen a large number of sex hormone-binding proteins can inhibit estrogen and its binding, reducing the biological activity of estrogen. Therefore, the phenomenon of menstrual disturbance is very important in female patients who take carbamazepine for a long time. In addition, enzyme-inducing drugs affect libido by reducing serum concentrations of total testosterone, free androgen index, DHEA sulfate, and estradiol. Topiramate and gabapentin have been reported to be associated with orgasmic disorder. However, women who comply with their antiepileptic medication prescriptions and have good seizure control may experience improved sexual function. In addition to their effect on sex hormones, liver enzyme-inducing drugs such as carbamazepine and phenytoin are also known to affect hormones such as thyroxine and triiodothyronine in both women and men. A meta-analysis of cross-sectional, case-control, and cohort studies evaluating the relationship between antiseizure medications and thyroid hormones found reduced concentrations of thyroxine (T4), free T4, and high thyrotropin in epileptic patients treated with antiseizure medications compared to healthy controls. Routine monitoring of thyroid function is not currently considered necessary in patients taking this class of drugs.

Enzyme-inhibiting antiseizure medications such as valproic acid significantly increase the risk of reproductive and sexual dysfunction. Valproic acid is associated with hyperandrogenism, insulin resistance, weight gain, polycystic ovaries, polycystic ovary syndrome, menstrual disorders, ovulation failure, and female infertility. Therefore, women who are fertile should try to avoid the use of valproate. When the use of valproate is needed to control seizures, the signs and symptoms should be regularly asked about by the attending physician and the patient should be referred to a gynecologist if necessary.

In addition to the effects of the above antiseizure medication types on sex hormones, there are also studies that show that combination antiseizure medication treatments are associated with more abnormal reproductive endocrine function than is monotherapy.

In recent years, the use of new antiseizure medications has gradually replaced the old generation of antiseizure medications. However, no studies have clearly shown that new antiseizure medications such as lamotrigine and levetiracetam have an effect on sex hormones and female endocrine function.

3.3 Catamenial Epilepsy

Ziyi Chen and Leihao Sha

3.3.1 Diagnosis and Treatment of Catamenial Epilepsy

Compared with male patients, female patients have special endocrine characteristics due to their menstrual cycle, and women also need to consider pregnancy, heredity, appearance and shape, among other things. Understanding the correlative mechanism driving the association between seizures and menstrual cycle would be helpful to develop treatment strategies for patients with catamenial epilepsy, timely warning of seizures, and strengthening prognostic management in order to improve the quality of life of patients.

3.3.1.1 Concept and Classification of Catamenial Epilepsy

Most epileptic seizures are not random. In more than 50% of cases, epileptic seizures are clustered. In addition, in a large proportion of male (29%) and female (35%) patients with epilepsy, epileptic seizures can be accompanied by chrono-rhythm. Following female puberty, rapid endocrine changes occur, the hypothalamic-pituitary-gonadal axis commences, progesterone is periodically secreted, menarche occurs, and the menstrual cycle is formed. The onset of the menstrual cycle is often accompanied by periodic fluctuations in the level of sex hormones, which will influence seizures. Studies have shown that from 3 days before menstruation to 3 days after menstruation, the level of progesterone drops sharply, which is associated with seizure induction. Estrogen reaches its peak level before ovulation, when the level of progesterone is low, the ratio of female progesterone is the highest, resulting in seizure aggravation. In the presence of pituitary insufficiency, progesterone levels are low and it is also easy to induce seizures. As mentioned above, when the periodicity of exacerbation of seizures in women with epilepsy coincides with the menstrual cycle, it is often referred to as catamenial epilepsy.

There remains no widely accepted, international definition of catamenial epilepsy, but according to the latest classifications such as that of Herzog, catamenial epilepsy can be divided into the following three types (Fig. 3.1):

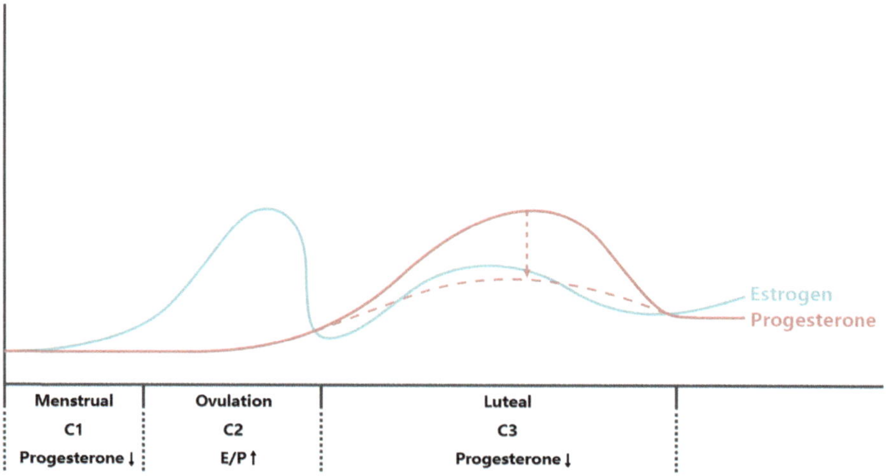

Fig. 3.1 Classification of catamenial epilepsy and its relationship with progesterone and estrogen. *C1* catamenial epilepsy type I, *C2* catamenial epilepsy type II, *C3* catamenial epilepsy type III, *E* estrogen, *P* progesterone

Menstrual period catamenial epilepsy (Type I): Characterized by increased frequency of seizures during the menstrual period (3 days before menstruation to 3 days after menstruation). The levels of progesterone and its metabolites in the premenstrual period decrease dramatically, the effect on gamma-aminobutyric acid decreases, and the excitability of neurons increases. Early clinical studies have shown water retention and neuronal cell swelling at the end of the luteal phase, increased excitability in animal models, and seizures in humans.

Ovulation catamenial epilepsy (Type II): An increase in the frequency of seizures during ovulation (10–13 days after menstruation) is characteristic. Estrogen levels peak during ovulation, while progesterone is at a relatively low level, and thus the estrogen/progesterone ratio (E/P) is highest, and seizures increase in frequency and severity. As estrogen levels decrease after ovulation, progesterone levels increase and E/P decreases, resulting in a reduced frequency and severity of seizures.

Luteal insufficiency catamenial epilepsy (Type III): Characterized by increased frequency of seizures during the menstrual cycle (ovulation, luteal, and menstrual periods) with luteal insufficiency. The patient has low serum progesterone levels, insufficient luteal function, and non-reflexive ovulation. Due to the lack of serum progesterone, which is insufficient to maintain the activity of gamma-aminobutyric acid neurons, the excitability of motor neurons in the cerebral cortex is elevated.

3.3.1.2 Diagnosis of Catamenial Epilepsy

The diagnosis of catamenial epilepsy consists of the following three steps: (1) the patient is diagnosed with epilepsy, (2) there is a clear history of menstruation-related seizures, and (3) categorization of the seizures experienced by the confirmed patients. Compared with the common types of epilepsy in clinical practice, the diagnosis of catamenial epilepsy is emphasized more on the patient's previous menstrual and seizure history, the determination of changes in serum hormone levels, the determination of changes in ASM serum concentrations, and other special examinations that are closely related to the pathogenesis of catamenial epilepsy.

Electroencephalogram examination also has a certain role in the diagnosis of catamenial epilepsy. Previous studies have reported that the incidence of catamenial epilepsy is higher in temporal lobe epilepsy, and seizures starting from the left temporal lobe are more common than those that start from the right. In the past, quantitative electroencephalogram (qEEG) changes in the ovarian cycle of patients with temporal lobe epilepsy were evaluated and analyzed, and the results showed that the decrease of menstrual α rhythm may be the cause of seizures in patients with type I temporal lobe epilepsy. This special qEEG pattern can be used as a biomarker of type I catamenial epilepsy and help to distinguish it from other types of catamenial epilepsy. Previous studies have also found differences in heart rate variability (HRV) in patients with different types of menstrual seizures. HRV is related to cardiac autonomic activity and can be used to assess autonomic control of the heart. Reduced HRV in women with a diagnosis of type I catamenial epilepsy helps to distinguish between the other two types of catamenial epilepsy.

3.3.2 The Role of Sex Hormones in Catamenial Epilepsy

At present, there is no uniform protocol for the treatment of catamenial epilepsy, and the general principle of treatment depends on whether the menstrual cycle is regular. Treatment options include medications and other treatments.

3.3.2.1 General Drug Treatment of Catamenial Epilepsy

General medical treatment for catamenial epilepsy includes ASMs, benzodiazepines, and acetazolamide. Regular ASMs are the mainstay of treatment, and the emphasis is on monotherapy over the course of treatment. However, the efficacy of ASMs is generally poor. Sodium valproate is the most commonly used class of nitrogen-free broad-spectrum antiseizure medications worldwide, but the toxic side effects in women with epilepsy are also more apparent, including polycystic ovary syndrome (PCOS), hypothalamic amenorrhea, premature menopause, and functional hyperprolactinemia. In 2018, the European Medicines Agency (EMA) adopted new restrictions on the administration of valproate to women of childbearing age and pregnant women, highlighting that valproate should only be used when there is no other suitable alternative medicine, and women of childbearing age should be strictly on contraceptive medication and use small doses of valproate. A number of new antiseizure medications have been used to demonstrate good outcomes for patients including those with catamenial epilepsy. Lamotrigine is a voltage-dependent sodium channel blocker that has a good antiepileptic effect and is often superior to other ASMs in stabilizing mood and restoring cognitive function. Lamotrigine and levetiracetam are recommended as the first choice for patients with fertility needs. Clobazam belongs to a new class of benzodiazepines that enhance the inhibitory effect of GABAergic neurons by binding to the BZD site on the GABAA receptor, thereby reducing anxiety symptoms and inhibiting seizures. In the 1980s, individual cases were reported of clobazam being used for the treatment of catamenial epilepsy with some success. More relevant medical evidence is needed in the future.

Acetazolamide is a carbonic anhydrase inhibitor that can effectively reduce the level of bicarbonate ions in brain cells, reduce ion outflow, and enhance the inhibition of GABAA receptors to reduce neuronal excitability; it is thus also used in the special drug treatment of catamenial epilepsy. Both daily continuous administration and use during the menstrual period are effective in alleviating seizures. Previous studies have shown that acetazolamide can reduce seizures by more than 50% in 40% of patients. There appears to be no significant difference in the effect of acetazolamide on general epilepsy, focal epilepsy, temporal lobe epilepsy, and extratemporal epilepsy, and no significant difference in the effect of continuous and intermittent medication use. However, in 15% of patients with catamenial epilepsy, acetazolamide therapy fails after 6–24 months.

3.3.2.2 Research Progress on the Role of Sex Hormones in Catamenial Epilepsy

Patients with catamenial epilepsy have obvious reproductive endocrine changes, and a large number of studies have shown that sex hormone therapy is effective for catamenial epilepsy. Estrogen has not been used in clinical experimental treatment of epilepsy due to its complex neuronal excitatory effects (both pro- and antiepileptic effects have been reported). However, progesterone has a sedative and anticonvulsant effect, so maintaining high progesterone levels during menstruation can help reduce seizures. Recent studies have shown that 31% of patients with catamenial epilepsy (especially types I and III) have worsening seizures related to decreased progesterone levels. A 3-year clinical observation study showed that periodic oral progesterone given to women with epilepsy was effective in a small number of women, and the frequency of seizures was reduced by more than 50% in post-hoc analysis, while the primary analysis failed to demonstrate efficacy. In addition, vaginal progesterone suppository use in the presence of frequent seizures can play a role in controlling menstrual seizures and can reduce the occurrence of adverse reactions. Studies have also shown that progesterone is effective for focal seizures. However, oral progesterone is associated with adverse reactions such as hot flushes and vaginal bleeding.

In addition, synthetic GnRH hormones such as triptorelin and goserelin have also been shown to play a role in the treatment of catamenial epilepsy. Neurosteroids are synthesized in glial cells from cholesterol through a series of enzymatic reactions, including progesterone, androgen, adrenal corticosteroids, and other derivatives. Under more than 20 years of professional research by Reddy et al., "neurosteroid replacement therapy (NRT)" was creatively proposed based on the mechanism of neurosteroid withdrawal (NSW), and it was found that neurosteroids or synthetic substances have strong anticonvulsant activity in animal models of catamenial epilepsy. Further observations found a significant gender difference in the antiepileptic activity of neurosteroids, with women more sensitive than men, which also has important significance for personalized neurosteroid replacement therapy for epileptic seizures. Ganaxolone is an allopregnanolone analogue, a serotonin receptor agonist that is well tolerated, has low drug interactions, and can be used well with ASMs. In a mouse model of catamenial epilepsy (type I), ganaxolone reduces the worsening of epilepsy. The drug is currently in phase II clinical trials in the United States. In addition, tetrahydroprogesterone and brexanolone are also currently popular neurosteroid products, which have potential for broad application in the field of catamenial epilepsy. At present, study of the role of progesterone supplement therapy in the treatment of female catamenial epilepsy is in progress abroad. Other hormonal therapies include the estrogen antagonist clomiphene and chorionic gonadotropin analogues, which may be effective but are poorly studied and carry a high risk of complications.

3.4 Hormone Therapy in Epilepsy

Leihao Sha

Epilepsy and seizures could be affected by sex hormones. Multiple studies investigated the different effects of hormones for patients with epilepsy to provide evidence for hormone therapy in epilepsy. Table 3.1 summarizes the effects of different hormones for epilepsy and seizures.

Table 3.1 Effects of hormones for seizures

Hormone	Name	Effect
Estrogen	Estradiol	1. Promote seizures and reduce electroshock threshold 2. Anticonvulsant
Progesterone	Progesterone, ganaxolone, long-acting medroxyprogesterone acetate, norethisterone, megestrol	Increased conduction of chloride ions, causing direct neuronal inhibition
	Pure natural progesterone vaginal pad, Prempro (0.625 mg combined equine estrogen +2.5 mg medroxyprogesterone acetate or CEE/MPA)	No effect
GnRH	Triptorelin, goserelin	Reduced production of FSH and LH, reduced seizures secondary to reduced production of LH and estrogen as a result of continued GnRH release
Testosterone	Testosterone	Converted into estrogen and 5alpha-reducing androgens, which affect seizures

3.4.1 Estrogen

The estrogen receptor is widely distributed throughout the brain and exerts its effects through non-genomic and genomic pathways. The non-genomic pathway takes effect within seconds and has a short duration, while the genomic pathway is slower to take effect and has a longer duration.

In animal experiments with rats, estrogen has been shown to have an excitatory effect on neurons, promoting firing and reducing the threshold for electroshock, as well as increasing the severity of chemically induced seizures.

1. This is thought to be secondary to a decrease in chloride ion conduction through the γ-aminobutyric acid (GABA) a receptor complex and inhibition of GABA (inhibitory central neurotransmitter) synthesis.
2. Estradiol also increases neuronal response to glutamate, an excitatory central neurotransmitter.
3. Although estrogen has been found to have pro-convulsant properties, it has also been found to have anti-convulsant effects. The dose, route of administration, chronic administration vs. acute administration, and type of estrogen can determine whether estrogen acts as a pro- or anti-convulsant agent.

3.4.2 Progesterone

Progesterone can increase the conduction of chloride ions, causing direct neuronal inhibition. This is largely the result of the action of a neuroactive metabolite of progesterone allopregnanolone. Progesterone primarily exhibits anti-convulsant properties through its metabolites, inhibiting firing and increasing the seizure threshold. In animals, progesterone has been shown to increase the threshold for electroshock and chemical-induced seizures. Research also suggests that women with menstrual epilepsy have lower serum progesterone levels than healthy control patients at a similar stage in the menstrual cycle. Table 3.2 demonstrated details of previous clinical study of progesterone therapy.

1. Allopregnanolone has a strong effect on the GABAA receptors in the central nervous system, similar to potent benzodiazepines, and is 1000 times stronger than phenobarbital.
2. It binds to different sites on the GABAA receptor than GABA, benzodiazepines, and barbiturates. It is therefore believed that inhibiting progesterone metabolism may even exacerbate seizures in a patient with menstrual irregularities, as reported in a previous case report.
   - Ganaxolone (synthetic tetrahydroprogesterone analogue)
   - The positive modulation of the GABAA receptor by allopregnanolone has anti-convulsant effects. Ganaxolone has been associated with lower side effects in existing clinical studies, with sedation being the commonest adverse reaction. Promising results have been achieved in phase 1 and 2 studies of ganaxolone in the treatment of infantile spasms, menstrual epilepsy in women, and refractory partial epilepsy in adults.
   - Long-acting medroxyprogesterone acetate (MPA)
   - Following 150 mg intramuscular injection for 6 months, a case became seizure-free.
   - Norethindrone (NET)
   - A 5 mg daily regimen for 6 months has been shown to reduce the frequency of seizures in patients with refractory menstrual epilepsy by 80%.
   - Megestrol (MA)
   - Taking 80 mg during the second half (days 15–25) of the menstrual cycle for 3 months can reduce the frequency of seizures in patients with refractory menstrual epilepsy by 80%.
   - Natural progesterone
   - Use between day 18 and day 28 of the menstrual cycle has been shown to be ineffective.
   - Prempro (0.625 mg combined equine estrogen +2.5 mg medroxyprogesterone acetate or CEE/MPA)
   - This has been shown to increase seizure frequency.

3.4.3 Gonadotropin-Releasing Hormone (GnRH) and Its Synthetic Analogues

Continuous non-pulsatile release of GnRH primarily causes the disappearance of the pituitary anterior lobe release of LH and FSH, resulting in anovulation. The reduction in FSH and LH production leads to a decrease in seizures secondary to

Table 3.2 Previous clinical study of progesterone therapy

Author	Medication	Regimens	Time[a]	Studied population	Type of seizure	ASMs	Primary outcomes	Effect
Motta et al. (2013)	P	50 mg Sublingual tablets 2 × 25 mg dose Days 16–25 of each cycle	17.69 ± 10.71	Catamenial epilepsy	CPS	CBZ, VPA, PHT or two medications	Decline in the frequency	63.07%
					GS			62.19%
					SPS			100%
					MS			46%
Herzog (1986)	P	200 mg Three times daily on days 14–28 of treatment cycles	3	Catamenial epilepsy	SGMS	CBZ, LEV, LTG, TPM, PHT	>50% average daily seizure reduction	13/33
					CPS			18/76
					SPS			14/34
				Refractory epilepsy	SGMS			7/33
					CPS			21/99
					SPS			19/45
Harden et al. (2006)	Pr	Single dose	3	Postmenopausal women with epilepsy	SPS	PMT, PHT, CBZ, TPM, LTG, LEV, GBP	Decline in the frequency	37.5%
					CPS			−12.5%
					GS			0
		Double dose			SPS	TPM, CBZ, TGB, VPA, CZP, PHT, CZP, GBP		−14.3%
					CPS			−42.9%
					GS			−14.3%
Ramanujam et al. (2016)	G	Vaginal pessaries between days 18 and 28 of menstrual cycle	6	A woman with recurrent catamenial status epilepticus	GTCS and AS	PB, CBZ, VPA, Vigabatrin, intravenous midazolam	Decline in the frequency	No effect
	MPA	150 mg intramuscular injection	6					Seizure free
	NET	5 mg twice a day	6					
Najafi et al. (2013)	MA	80 mg in the second half of the cycle from 15th to 25th day	3	Intractable catamenial epilepsy	CPS	/	Decline in the frequency	80%
					SGS			
					PGS			

Dana-Haeri and Richens (1983)	NET	5 mg or 350 pg three times daily	12	Catamenial epilepsy	TCS CPS or SPS	/	Decline in the frequency	No effect
Bäckström et al. (1984)	P	Priming 0.5–3.0 mg of progesterone and continuous 4.0–12.0 mg/h of progesterone infusion	2 h	Catamenial epilepsy	PS	DPH, PB, CBZ, mephenytoin, PMT and CZP	Epileptic spike frequency	4/7 reduce 2/7 no change 1/7 increase
Davis et al. (2016)	P	IUD	6	Epilepsy	GT CS MS AS CPS	LTG, LEV, OXC, CBZ, LCM, VPA, CZP, TPM	Seizure number	3/20 worse 13/20 no change 4/20 improved

[a] Duration of medication (month). / information not available, *P* progesterone, *Pr* Prempro (0.625 mg of conjugated equine estrogens plus 2.5 mg of medroxyprogesterone acetate or CEE/MPA), *G* gesterone, *MPA* depot medroxyprogesterone, *NET* norethisterone, *MA* megestrol, *PS* partial seizure, *CPS* complex partial seizure, *SPS* simple partial seizure, *GS* generalized seizure, *PGS* primary generalized seizure, *SGS* secondary generalized seizure, *MS* myoclonic seizure, *SGMS* secondary generalized motor seizures, *AS* absence seizure, *GTCS* generalized tonic-clonic seizure, *TCS* tonic-clonic seizure, *ASMs* antiepileptic drugs, *CBZ* carbamazepine, *VPA* valproate, *PHT* phenytoin, *LEV* levetiracetam, *LTG* lamotrigine, *TPM* topiramate, *PMT* primidone, *GBP* gabapentin, *TGB* tiagabine, *CZP* clonazepam, *PB* phenobarbital, *DPH* diphenylhydantoin, *OXC* oxcarbazepine, *LCM* lacosamide

reduced LH and estrogen production caused by the continuous release of GnRH. Due to the cyclical changes in estrogen caused by GnRH, further research is needed to reduce seizure frequency before assessing the benefits and risks of using GnRH analogs to treat refractory epilepsy.

- Triptorelin
- The GnRH analog triptorelin was studied in ten women with refractory menstrual epilepsy and amenorrhea. It was administered by controlled-release depot formulation intramuscular injection, and the results indicated that three women reported no seizures, and four others reported a reduction in seizure frequency. This may be secondary to reduced LH and estrogen production caused by the continuous release of GnRH.
- Goserelin
- Goserelin was studied in a woman with recurrent menstrual epilepsy. It was found that after subcutaneous administration of goserelin every 4 weeks, the patient's hospital admissions for status epilepticus decreased.

3.4.4 Testosterone

Androgens are converted into estrogen and 5α-reducing androgens in the body, and estrogen has a convulsion-promoting function. Recent studies have shown that blocking the conversion of testosterone to estrogen through the use of aromatase inhibitors raises the seizure threshold, suggesting that lower testosterone levels and/or higher estradiol levels may be directly related to sexual dysfunction and increased seizure frequency in men with epilepsy. Chronically low testosterone can lead to testicular failure and hypergonadotropic hypogonadism, both of which are seen in men with epilepsy. In men with hypogonadism, testosterone normalization can significantly improve libido and sexual function. Therefore, for men with epilepsy who complain of sexual dysfunction, testosterone levels should be monitored, and testosterone supplementation may help improve sexual function, improve mood, and reduce seizure frequency.

3.4.5 Experience of Hormone Therapy in Epilepsy

Here, we would like to share our experience of hormone therapy (LNG-IUD) for refractory epilepsy in a female patient in West China Hospital of Sichuan University. The 38-year-old woman initially had a focal impaired awareness seizure, marked by limb convulsions and urinary incontinence, following a mental attack 12 years ago. She experienced aura such as daze, fear, anxiety, and occasional numbness throughout her body. These were followed by loss of consciousness, gripped hands, slight forearm flexion, movement, slurred speech, and occasional signs of stiff clenching of hands, without clonus. Each episode, occurring 1–2 times per month, lasted several minutes. Four years ago, she started experiencing nocturnal attacks with urinary incontinence during the latter half of her menstrual cycle without an apparent trigger. The frequent nocturnal episodes disrupted her sleep, causing her daytime mental well-being to worsen. All of those conditions seriously affected the life quality of her and her family. She was diagnosed with focal epilepsy with focal impaired awareness seizures and underwent evaluations. She took 24-h-video electroencephalography (24 h-VEEG) at that time. The background EEG displayed periods of normal activity with intermittent focal slowing noted. Photic stimulation revealed no seizure. And ictal findings showed electrographic correlate observed during seizures, characterized by rhythmic spikes evolving into sharp waves localized. Correlation with video recordings confirmed that electrographic changes corresponded temporally with observed clinical seizures, supporting the diagnosis of focal impaired awareness epilepsy. Magnetic resonance imaging (MRI) scans were considered negative 5 months ago. The patient could not recall the initial medication. Despite switching to Levetiracetam (1500 mg bid), Oxcarbazepine (750 mg tid), and Lacosamide (100 mg bid) when monotherapy proved ineffective, the new regimen also failed. Subsequently, she received a diagnosis of refractory epilepsy. She did not improve after taking the medicine and fell into a state of anxiety and depression. As her seizures became more frequent and her mood increasingly depressed and anxious, her overall condition deteriorated. Three years ago, to better control her seizures, Lacosamide was discontinued while Levetiracetam (1500 mg bid) and Oxcarbazepine (750 mg tid) were maintained.

Upon carefully reviewing the medical history, it was found that she had her first period at the age of 11 years and has been experiencing irregular vaginal bleeding since then. She was presented to a gynecologist for treatment to address the issue of irregular vaginal bleeding. Then, she was diagnosed with anovulatory dysfunctional uterine bleeding. To treat her irregular vaginal bleeding, the gynecologist offered a number of treatment options. She was given LNG IUD for treatment.

She presented to our hospital after undergoing intrauterine placement of LNG-IUD for 6 months. Following the treatment with LNG-IUD, she noted a gradual reduction in irregular bleeding. Moreover, she reported experiencing only one seizure, and there were no alterations made to the prescription of ASMs. During this period, she reported relaxed mood and maintained mental well-being. Subsequent follow-ups have revealed no further episodes, which means that LNG-IUD, the device had been placed to stop her irregular vaginal bleeding, accidentally cured the epilepsy that has plagued her for years. It prompted us to delve into profound considerations regarding the clinical treatment of individuals with refractory epilepsy. The patient's condition of seizures over time is shown in Fig. 3.2.

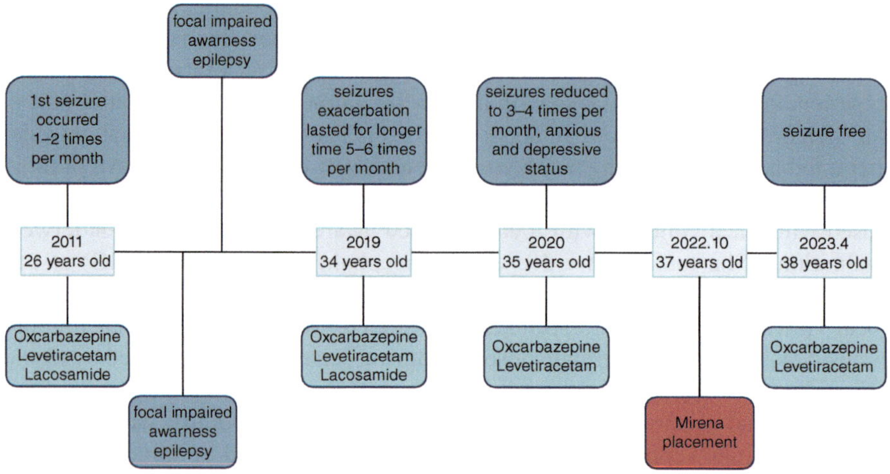

Fig. 3.2 Changes in the patient's seizures over time

References

Bäckström T, Zetterlund B, Blom S, et al. Effects of intravenous progesterone infusions on the epileptic discharge frequency in women with partial epilepsy. Acta Neurol Scand. 1984;69(4):240–8.

Dana-Haeri J, Richens A. Effect of norethisterone on seizures associated with menstruation. Epilepsia. 1983;24(3):377–81.

Davis AR, Saadatmand HJ, Pack A. Women with epilepsy initiating a progestin IUD: a prospective pilot study of safety and acceptability. Epilepsia. 2016;57(11):1843–8.

Harden CL, Herzog AG, Nikolov BG, et al. Hormone replacement therapy in women with epilepsy: a randomized, double-blind, placebo-controlled study. Epilepsia. 2006;47(9):1447–51.

Herzog AG. Intermittent progesterone therapy and frequency of complex partial seizures in women with menstrual disorders. Neurology. 1986;36(12):1607–10.

Motta E, Golba A, Ostrowska Z, et al. Progesterone therapy in women with epilepsy. Pharmacol Rep. 2013;65(1):89–98.

Najafi M, Sadeghi MM, Mehvari J, et al. Progesterone therapy in women with intractable catamenial epilepsy. Adv Biomed Res. 2013;2:8.

Ramanujam B, Arora A, Malhotra V, et al. A case of recurrent status epilepticus and successful management with progesterone. Epileptic Disord. 2016;18(1):101–5.

Suggested Readings

Bauer J, Wildt L, Flügel D, et al. The effect of a synthetic GnRH analogue on catamenial epilepsy: a study in ten patients. J Neurol. 1992;239(5):284–6.

Fu L. Sex hormones and catamenial epilepsy. Chin J Pract Med. 2008;14:141–3.

Haider Y, Barnett DB. Catamenial epilepsy and goserelin. Lancet. 1991;338(8781):1530.

Hamed SA. Neuroendocrine hormonal conditions in epilepsy: relationship to reproductive and sexual functions. Neurologist. 2008;14(3):157–69.

Herzog AG. Catamenial epilepsy: definition, prevalence pathophysiology and treatment. Seizure. 2008;17(2):151–9.

Herzog AG, Friedman MN. Menstrual cycle interval and ovulation in women with localization-related epilepsy. Neurology. 2001;57(11):2133–5.

Herzog AG, Seibel MM, Schomer DL, et al. Reproductive endocrine disorders in women with partial seizures of temporal lobe origin. Arch Neurol. 1986;43(4):341–6.

Herzog AG, Klein P, Jacobs AR. Testosterone versus testosterone and testolactone in treating reproductive and sexual dysfunction in men with epilepsy and hypogonadism. Neurology. 1998;50(3):782–4.

Herzog AG, Coleman AE, Jacobs AR, et al. Relationship of sexual dysfunction to epilepsy laterality and reproductive hormone levels in women. Epilepsy Behav. 2003;4(4):407–13.

Herzog AG, Harden CL, Liporace J, et al. Frequency of catamenial seizure exacerbation in women with localization-related epilepsy. Ann Neurol. 2004;56(3):431–4.

Laxer K, Blum D, Abou-Khalil BW, et al. Assessment of ganaxolone's anticonvulsant activity using a randomized, double-blind, presurgical trial design. Ganaxolone Presurgical Study Group. Epilepsia. 2000;41(9):1187–94.

Morris GL III, Vanderkolk C. Human sexuality, sex hormones, and epilepsy. Epilepsy Behav. 2005;7(Suppl 2):S22–8.

Reddy DS. The role of neurosteroids in the pathophysiology and treatment of catamenial epilepsy. Epilepsy Res. 2009;85(1):1–30.

Svalheim S, Sveberg L, Mochol M, et al. Interactions between antiepileptic drugs and hormones. Seizure. 2015;28:12–7.

Taubøll E, Sveberg L, Svalheim S. Interactions between hormones and epilepsy. Seizure. 2015;28:3–11.

Thomas SV, Sarma P, Nirmala C, et al. Women with epilepsy and infertility have different reproductive hormone profile than others. Ann Indian Acad Neurol. 2013;16(4):544–8.

Preconception Management of Women with Epilepsy

4

Ziyi Chen, Leihao Sha, and Lei Chen

4.1 Contraception in Women with Epilepsy

Ziyi Chen

4.1.1 Pregnancy Status and Contraception in Women with Epilepsy

Due to the effects of epilepsy and ASMs, fertility and pregnancy planning are affected in women with epilepsy. There have been conflicting data on fertility rates in women with epilepsy, however, most studies have shown a lower fertility rate in WWE. The Epilepsy Birth Control Registry (EBCR) group retrospectively examined the reproductive history of nearly 1000 WWE to assess infertility (no pregnancy after more than 1 year of not using contraception) and impaired fertility (percentage of women who were infertile or did not give birth to a live generation) and found an infertility rate of 9.2% and impaired fertility rate of 20.7% in WWE; these are higher than the rates in the general population (6.5% and 12.7%, respectively) (Herzog et al. 2016).

In addition, in order to avoid seizures and the adverse effects that ASMs may have on the mother and offspring, most WWE of childbearing age choose various forms of contraception to prevent unwanted pregnancies before planning a

Z. Chen
Department of Neurology, The First Affiliated Hospital, Sun Yat-sen University, Guangzhou, China
e-mail: chenziyi@mail.sysu.edu.cn

L. Sha · L. Chen (✉)
Department of Neurology, West China Hospital, Sichuan University, Chengdu, China

L. Chen (ed.), *Women with Epilepsy in Child-bearing Age*,
https://doi.org/10.1007/978-981-97-3921-9_4

pregnancy. Unfortunately, however, unplanned pregnancies are not uncommon in WWE. A recent EBCR study showed that nearly 60% of people with epilepsy are at risk of an unintended pregnancy. Nearly 30% of them were not using a highly effective method of birth control, and another 7% were using hormonal birth control along with enzyme-inducing antiseizure medications, putting them at risk of birth control failure. Contraceptive counseling is an important aspect of treatment for WWE. Regular hormonal contraceptives are highly effective, but there is a complex interaction between ASMs and hormonal contraceptives that may be responsible for contraceptive failure and/or poor seizure control. However, most WWE who take enzyme-inducing ASMs do not have a good understanding of the interactions between medications and hormonal contraceptives, and many clinicians still do not have a good understanding of WWE contraception during the reproductive age, resulting in a low percentage of WWE users who receive contraceptive counseling and use the correct contraceptive method. The U.S. Epilepsy Birth Control Registry surveyed contraceptive practices in the community among 1144 WWE, finding that 87.2% had been seen by a neurologist but only 25.4% had received professional contraception counseling. Therefore, an important task in the management of WWE is to understand the fertility status and pregnancy risks of WWE and choose the appropriate contraceptive methods.

4.1.2 Contraceptive Risks in Women with Epilepsy

Common methods of contraception for women include hormonal and non-hormonal contraception. Hormonal contraceptive methods include: (1) combined hormonal contraceptive methods: combined oral contraceptives (COCs), combined hormonal skin patch, and vaginal ring; (2) progesterone contraceptive methods: oral tablets (POPs) containing progesterone only, subcutaneous implantations of progesterone, progesterone long-acting contraceptive injections, and uterine IUDs releasing progesterone; and (3) emergency contraceptive pills. Non-hormonal contraceptive methods include: contraceptive barriers, copper IUDs, ligation, and safe period contraceptive methods. Adherence to different forms of birth control varies greatly. Studies have reported that hormonal contraceptives were the most frequently discontinued form of WWE during the reproductive age (50.7%), and IUD was the least discontinued form of contraception (25.1%). The top three reasons for discontinuation were poor contraceptive reliability (13.9%), menstrual disorders (13.5%), and increased seizures (8.6%) (Reddy 2017).

4.1.2.1 Interplay Between Hormonal Contraception and ASMs

The biological transformation process ASMs undergo in the body can influence the effects of biological enzymes such as CYP450 and UGT. ASMs can be divided into the following categories based on the biological metabolic effects that ASMs have on CYP450 and UGT: (1) enzyme-inducing AEDs (EIAEDs), which include phenobarbital, phenytoin, carbamazepine, oxcarbazepine, perampanel, and topiramate (dose >200 mg/day); (2) non-enzyme-inducing AEDs (NEIAEDs), including levetiracetam, zonisamide, gabapentin, lacosamide, pregabalin, tiagabine, and topiramate (dose ≤200 mg/day); (3) GluAEDs (GluAEDs), including lamotrigine only; (4) enzyme-inhibitor AEDs (InhAEDs), including only valproate. In addition, lamotrigine also belongs to the EIAEDs group, but its degree of enzyme induction is weaker than other EIAEDs.

On the one hand, the administration of EIAEDs can stimulate the expression of CYP450 and UGT, accelerate the metabolism of estrogen and progesterone, and reduce its serum concentration. On the other hand, blood sex hormone-binding globulin (SHBG) can be significantly increased, reducing the concentration of free and bioactive endogenous or exogenous steroids in the body. In conclusion, EIAEDs can reduce the contraceptive effect of COCs, complex hormone skin patch, complex hormone vaginal ring, POPs, progesterone subcutaneous implantation, and other contraceptive methods, leading to unintended pregnancy. Even if the dosage of oral contraceptives is increased during the regular medication cycle, there is no guarantee that the effective contraceptive effect will be maintained while taking EIAEDs. For this reason, neither the Centers for Disease Control and Prevention (CDC) nor the World Health Organization (WHO) recommend using EIAEDs in combination with oral hormonal contraceptives, vaginal rings, or transdermal patches.

Carbamazepine, phenytoin, and phenobarbital belong to a broad spectrum of enzyme inducers that induce large amounts of CYP450 and UGT production, thereby accelerating the metabolism of estrone. However, the new generation of drugs oxcarbazepine, rufinamide, topiramate (dose >200 mg/day), and perampanel (dose ≥8 mg/day) have relatively weak enzyme inducibility and can only stimulate the production of limited CYP450 and UGT. Progesterone tablets in emergency contraceptives are also affected by EIAEDs, but copper-containing IUDs are not affected by ASMs. Although there is little evidence of an interaction between ASMs and POPs, EIAEDs, like estrogen, also increase the metabolism of progesterone, so the effectiveness of POPs and EIAEDs is reduced when used in combination, but intradermal injections of long-acting medroxyprogesterone and levonorgestrel-releasing IUD are not affected by ASMs.

4.1.2.2 Effects of Hormonal Contraceptives on Specific ASMs

While ASMs accelerate female and progesterone metabolism and reduce the effectiveness of hormonal contraceptives, estrogen itself can also affect the metabolism of other drugs and serum concentrations by inhibiting cytochrome enzymes and inducing UGT enzymes. Therefore, hormonal contraceptives may also have an impact on the efficacy of certain ASMs. COCs can induce the UGT system thereby increasing the metabolism of drugs such as lamotrigine through glucosylation. Studies have shown that the combination of lamotrigine and estrogen-containing hormonal contraceptives (including oral formulations, vaginal rings, and skin patches) accelerates the glucogenation process, which in turn decreases serum concentrations of lamotrigine by more than 50%, ultimately leading to an increase in the frequency or recurrence of seizures. Progesterone contraceptives do not alter serum levels of lamotrigine, although estrogen has a strong effect on lamotrigine. Hormonal contraceptives also reduce serum valproic acid concentration through a similar mechanism of action, but the degree of reduction is not significant. In addition, hormonal contraceptives may affect oxcarbazepine in a similar manner because its active metabolite ricamazepine (monohydroxy-carbamazepine) is also metabolized by gluconylation.

4.1.2.3 Effects of Contraceptive Pills on Seizure Control

Estrogen is associated with neuroexcitability and can lower the seizure threshold, while progesterone has anti-epileptic effects through the metabolite medroxyprogesterone, so the use of hormonal contraceptives may affect neuronal excitability and seizure threshold. The widespread use of hormonal contraceptives has also had an impact on the control of WWE seizures in the childbearing years. Studies have shown that different types of contraception have different effects on seizures during the reproductive age in WWE, and that for patients who take hormonal contraceptives with any ASMs, the increased probability of seizures is higher than that associated with non-hormonal contraceptives. Among hormonal contraceptives, complex hormonal patches and subcutaneous implantation of progesterone have the highest probability of being associated with increased seizures, while long-acting medroxyprogesterone has a higher probability of being associated with reduced seizures than combined hormonal contraceptives. When exposed to estrogens as part of COP or postmenopausal hormone replacement therapy, the blood levels of lamotrigine were observed to decrease by 50%. In addition, NEIAEDs was associated with the least increased probability of seizures when hormonal contraceptives were used. The probability of increased seizures may be higher when hormonal contraceptives are used with other ASMs.

4.1.3 Contraceptive Methods for Women with Epilepsy

Given the complex interactions between hormonal contraceptives and ASMs, combined use may reduce the effectiveness of both simultaneously; thus, choosing the right contraceptive method is important for WWE of childbearing age (Table 4.1).

For WWE of childbearing age taking EIAEDs, medroxyprogesterone acetate long-acting injections, levonorgestrel release IUDs, and copper-containing IUDs are not affected by EIAEDs and can be used as the primary contraceptive method. Medroxyprogesterone acetate intradermal injection is a long-acting reversible contraceptive method that can be used together with EIAEDs. Its progesterone concentration and contraceptive efficacy are high, but it can affect the peak bone value before the age of 20 years, leading to a risk of bone mineral density loss, so it is not a first-line choice. The failure rate of IUD contraceptive devices is 0.2–0.8% per year, which is significantly lower than that of commonly used hormonal or non-hormonal contraceptive methods. Previous preclinical studies have shown that progestogen-containing IUDs are a safe and long-acting contraceptive method. Therefore, IUDs may be the best choice for patients. In addition, the Royal College of Obstetricians and Gynaecologists in the United Kingdom recommends that an intrauterine copper IUD be inserted as emergency contraception for women taking

Table 4.1 Effectiveness and recommended methods of hormonal contraceptive use in WWE during childbearing age

Hormonal contraceptive methods	Unintended pregnancy rates in the USA/year	ASM impact	Recommended forms of birth control
Combined hormonal birth control			When used with EIAEDs, it should be replaced with a copper-containing IUD or levonorgestrel IUD or an intramural medroxyprogesterone acetate; oral hormone complexes containing high doses of ethinylestradiol may be considered for continuous administration
COCs	9%	Affected by EIAEDs, reduced efficacy	
Compound hormonal skin patches	9%	Affected by EIAEDs, reduced efficacy	
Complex hormonal vaginal ring	9%	Affected by EIAEDs, reduced efficacy	
Progesterone method of contraception			When used with EIAEDs, it should be replaced with a copper-containing IUD or levonorgestrel IUD or an intramural medroxyprogesterone acetate
POPs	9%	Affected by EIAEDs, reduced efficacy	
Etonogestrel is implanted subcutaneously	0.05%	May be affected by EIAEDs, reducing efficacy	
Progesterone long-acting contraceptive shots	6%	Not affected by EIAEDs	
IUD	<1%	Not affected by EIAEDs	

(continued)

Table 4.1 (continued)

Hormonal contraceptive methods	Unintended pregnancy rates in the USA/year	ASM impact	Recommended forms of birth control
Emergency contraceptive pills			Copper-based IUDs are recommended, or emergency contraceptive tablets with a 2× dose of progesterone
Oral progesterone tablets	9%	Affected by EIAEDs, reduced efficacy	
Copper containing IUD	<1%	Not affected by EIAEDs	

EIAEDs when needed, or that emergency contraception tablets with progesterone be taken at a 2× (3 mg) dose. If intramuscular medroxyprogesterone acetate, IUD, and other options are not acceptable to the patient, it is recommended to consider COCs containing high doses of ethinylestradiol (50–60 g) in a continuous manner or in a triple cycle. The triple cycle refers to the continuous use of three to four cycles of hormonal contraceptives prior to a 4-day pill-free interval before continuing to take the pill, following which the same schedule repeats. However, there is no evidence to support this recommendation. Therefore, additional barrier contraception is also recommended for patients using COCs. For WWE of childbearing age taking NEIAEDs, any available method of contraception may be appropriate.

Clinicians should make a point of offering contraceptive counseling from the initial patient visit. Patients with epilepsy who are not taking EIAEDs should also be informed of this interaction, as the treatment regimen for future patients may shift to EIAEDs. Conversely, if there is a switch from EIAEDs to NEIAEDs, then the dosage of hormonal contraceptives needs to be adjusted so as to avoid adverse reactions caused by drug overdose.

4.2 Epilepsy and Polycystic Ovary Syndrome

Leihao Sha and Ziyi Chen

4.2.1 The Relationship Between Epilepsy, Antiseizure Medications, and Polycystic Ovary Syndrome

For women with epilepsy, the main diseases related to reproductive dysfunction caused by epilepsy include: polycystic ovary syndrome (PCOS), amenorrhea, menstrual disorders, premature ovarian failure, and low ovarian function. In recent years, PCOS has attracted extensive attention in the study of women with epilepsy because of its great harm, and it is one of the most important causes of anovulation infertility (Verrotti et al. 2011).

4.2.1.1 Overview of Polycystic Ovary Syndrome

PCOS is the commonest gynecological endocrine disorder in women of childbearing age, affecting more than 10% of the total population of women. The typical characteristics of PCOS include irregular menstruation, hirsute (Fig. 4.1), acne, obesity, and infertility. It has become the main cause of ovulation disorder and infertility in women of childbearing age. Modern medicine postulates that PCOS is a disease caused by multi-factor and multi-gene interactions, and the disease has the characteristics of heredity and family aggregation. In the onset and progression of PCOS, obesity, insulin resistance, life, psycho-psychological factors, inflammatory response, hyperandrogenism, and other factors all play a promoting role. The diagnostic criteria for PCOS are as follows:

1. Diagnosis of PCOS during reproductive age and perimenopause
   (a) Suspected PCOS: Irregular menstruation or amenorrhea or irregular uterine bleeding is a necessary condition for diagnosis. In addition, one of the following two conditions should be met: (1) hyperandrogenic clinical

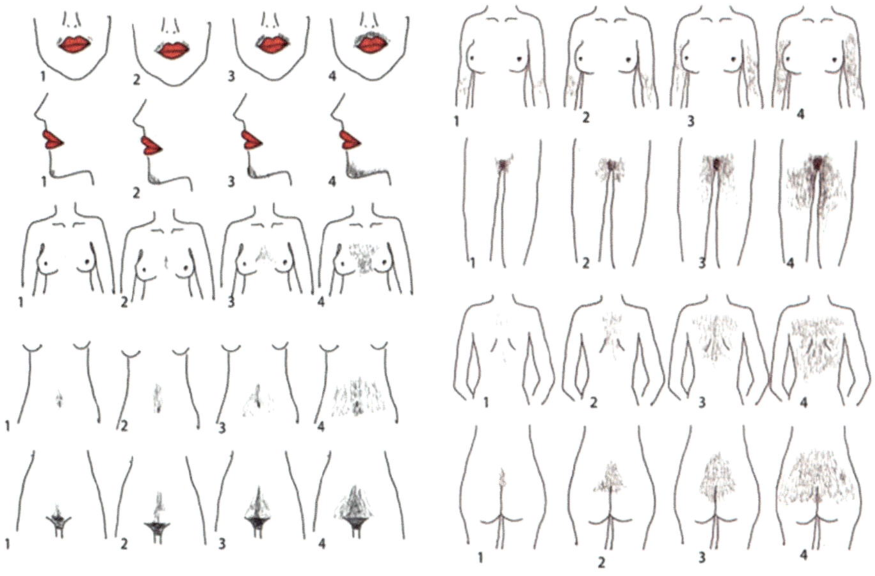

Fig. 4.1 Assessment of hirsutism (Ferryman and Gallwey Rating). The nine sites sensitive to androgen were upper lip, chin, chest, upper abdomen, lower abdomen, upper back, lower back, upper arm, and thigh, which were divided into four grades (1–4) according to the severity of hirsutism. The total score of each site was added to the F-G score, and the total score ≥8 points indicated hirsutism

manifestations or hyperandrogenemia and (2) polycystic ovary morphology on ultrasound.

(b) Diagnosis of PCOS: After the above diagnostic criteria for suspected PCOS are met, other diseases that may cause hyperandrogenism and cause abnormal ovulation must be individually excluded before the diagnosis of PCOS can be confirmed.

2. The diagnosis of PCOS in adolescence

   The diagnosis of PCOS in adolescence must meet all three of the following criteria: (1) sporadic menstruation lasting at least 2 years after menarche or amenorrhea, (2) hyperandrogenic clinical manifestations or hyperandrogenemia, and (3) ovarian PCOM manifestations under ultrasound.
3. Other diseases with high androgen manifestations, such as primary adrenal hyperplasia, androgen-secreting tumors, and Cushing syndrome should be excluded.

PCOS profoundly affects patients' quality of life, with a high risk of infertility, obesity, and other metabolic disorders. It is estimated that patients with PCOS have a 3.26 times risk of impaired glucose tolerance and 2.87 times risk of type 2 diabetes mellitus. PCOS is also a common cause of anovulation and a risk factor for endometrial cancer. Furthermore, PCOS could cause potential damage to brain function. Lai et al. reported impaired function in multiple brain regions of PCOS patients including the left inferior temporal gyrus, left inferior occipital gyrus, and superior frontal gyrus, which are associated with visuospatial working memory, face processing, and episodic memory (Lai et al. 2020). These changes are also related to sex hormones including luteinizing hormone. And altered brain network connectivity is observed for patients with both epilepsy and PCOS, which indicated the interaction effect of epilepsy of PCOS on brain activity (Figs. 4.2 and 4.3). Such evidence could indicate that the links between PCOS and the brain could be associated with the hypothalamic-pituitary-gonadal axis, as previous research reported that altered levels of hormones could affect the function of the brain.

4.2.1.2 PCOS and Epilepsy

The incidence of PCOS in the general population is 8–13%, but the incidence of PCOS in patients with epilepsy is approximately 10.5–26%, indicating that the incidence of PCOS is higher (approximately double) in patients with epilepsy than in the general population. At present, most scholars believe that the occurrence of PCOS in epilepsy patients is not only related to epilepsy but also to ASMs, especially valproic acid. Research has shown that the occurrence of epilepsy and the pharmacological action of antiseizure medications can target certain substrates, affect hormone levels, and cause disorders of the reproductive endocrine and metabolic system, including the limbic system, liver, hypothalamus, pituitary gland, ovaries, and adipose tissue.

A possible link between epilepsy and PCOS was first proposed in 1984, and studies in recent years have shown that WWE are more likely to develop PCOS than women who do not have epilepsy. In addition, several other studies on reproductive

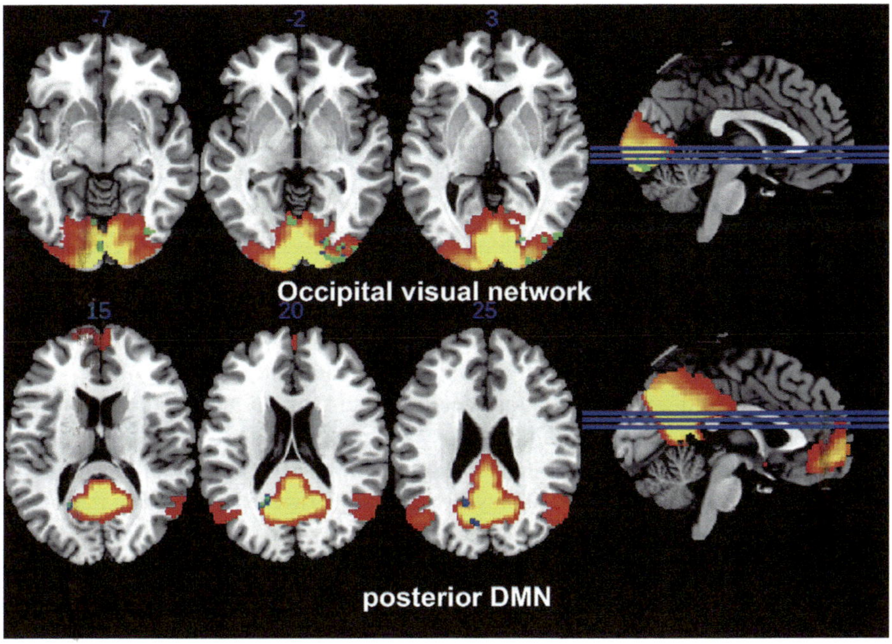

Fig. 4.2 Interactions of epilepsy and PCOS on brain intra-network connectivity in women with epilepsy and PCOS. *DMN* default mode network

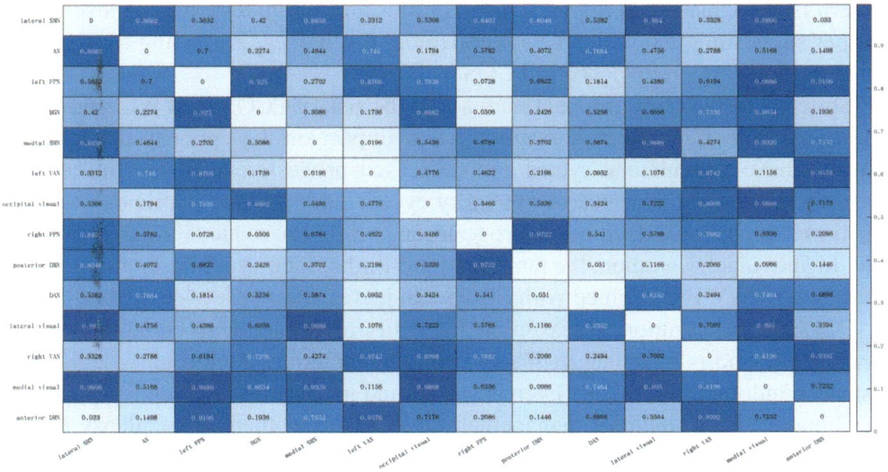

Fig. 4.3 Interaction effects between epilepsy and PCOS on connections between different resting brain networks. The value represents the $(1 - p)$ value, and the darker the blue, the larger the $(1 - p)$ value. *SMN* sensorimotor network, *AN* auditory network, *BGN* basal ganglia network, *FPN* frontal parietal network, *VAN* ventral attention network, *DAN* dorsal attention network, *DMN* default mode network

endocrine disorders in patients with epilepsy have also confirmed that epilepsy may increase the harm of reproductive endocrine disorders in WWE, making WWE more susceptible to altered hormone levels, abnormal menstrual cycles, polycystic ovaries, and PCOS. Previous studies have shown that epileptic discharges act on some hypothalamic structures that produce, secrete, and regulate GnRH, such as the arcoid nucleus and paraventricular nucleus, to increase the frequency or amplitude of GnRH pulses, thereby enhancing LH pulse release and increasing the LH/FSH ratio, which leads to abnormal hormone secretion levels in the HPO axis, ultimately leading to the development of PCOS. In addition, studies have shown that seizures in the limbic lobe may simultaneously decrease plasma dopamine levels, resulting in elevated LH and increased pituitary prolactin release, increasing the risk of PCOS. Patients with epilepsy and reproductive endocrine disorders often present with neurotransmitter dysfunction or genetic defects, which may also play a role in the association between PCOS and epilepsy.

The incidence of PCOS has been shown to be related to the age of onset of epilepsy, but not to the type or frequency of seizures. However, there have been conflicting studies regarding the relationship between seizure type and PCOS, with studies suggesting that PCOS is more common in focal epilepsy, especially left temporal lobe epilepsy (TLE). TLE is one of the commonest types of epilepsy in women of childbearing age, and a large amount of PCOS research has focused on people with TLE. On the other hand, this is attributed to the fact that the structure of the temporal lobe is closely connected to the hypothalamic anatomy, and the fibrous connections are extensive and direct. Studies based on animal models have shown that TLE is strongly associated with higher pulse frequency GnRH secretion, which in turn is associated with higher LH/FSH ratios and serum testosterone levels, thus further suggesting that patients with epileptoid discharges originating from the left temporal lobe are predisposed to PCOS.

Epilepsy leads to a significant increase in the risk of PCOS in WWE, and WWE combined with PCOS also has a significant impact on the epilepsy itself. PCOS patients have anovulatory cycles and decreased progesterone levels, and studies have shown that the absence of ovulatory cycles can trigger epileptic discharge in the limbic lobe, and a decrease in progesterone levels can reduce the seizure threshold. In anovulatory women, the temporal lobe-limbic lobe structures are sensitive to estrogen, so WWE combined with PCOS can increase the risk of seizures.

PCOS is the commonest reason for infertility of women with epilepsy of childbearing age and is associated with several risks including altered glucose metabolism and endometrial cancer. Given its harms and interactions with epilepsy, experts in China recommend closer management of PCOS in women with epilepsy including early prevention, early diagnosis, and early treatment. All women with epilepsy in pre-adulthood and of reproductive age should avoid the use of valproic acid and conduct standard diagnostic procedures for PCOS. The most highly recommended diagnostic criteria for PCOS is the Rotterdam criteria, proposed by the European Society of Human Reproduction and Embryology and the American Society of Reproductive Medicine in 2003. The definition proposes that PCOS can be diagnosed in any woman presenting with at least two of the three following characteristics: clinical and/or biochemical hyperandrogenism, ovulatory dysfunction, and PCOM, along with the exclusion of specific disorders with similar symptoms, such as hyperprolactinemia, thyroid dysfunction, and androgen-secreting tumors. However, many scholars and clinicians have argued that PCOS is overdiagnosed by the Rotterdam criteria as they incorporate androgen excess, which is not a vital indicator. As a major comorbidity of women with epilepsy, PCOS should be recognized and managed earlier. The Rotterdam criteria are applicable in clinical practice, but should not be used as a large-scale screening tool. Lai et al. reported different characteristics of women with epilepsy who have PCOS compared with those who do not have PCOS. They suggested patients with epilepsy and PCOS are of younger age at the onset of epilepsy, have a history of hypoxia at birth, higher luteinizing hormone levels, and other signs. A predictive model with an area under the curve (AUC) of 0.931 was established for better recognition of PCOS in women with epilepsy.

4.2.1.3 PCOS and Antiseizure Medications

There is a growing body of research exploring the correlation between ASMs and PCOS. In addition to valproic acid (VPA), the correlation between ASMs and PCOS is also receiving increasing attention. Previous studies on the effects of VPA on ovarian androgen production have shown that VPA can promote ovarian androgen biosynthesis, cause chromatin variation, and thus increase the replication of steroid-producing genes. These studies provide evidence in support of VPA-induced PCOS, establishing a direct correlation between valproate therapy and increased ovarian androgen biosynthesis. In a number of subsequent studies examining the association between antiseizure medications and PCOS, the results showed that PCO-like lesions, hyperandrogenemia, ovulation dysfunction, and menstrual disorders were more common in women taking VPA for epilepsy than in those who did not take VPA and those who took other ASMs, further suggesting a relationship between VPA and PCOS.

The reason for the increase in the incidence of PCOS caused by VPA is unknown. The possible factors are: (1) VPA increases the release of GABA in the central nervous system, which may affect the pulsatile release of gonadotropin; (2) VPA leads to increased body mass and weight gain is likely to lead to insulin resistance and hyperinsulinemia, which may be a key factor in the pathogenesis of PCOS; (3) the pharmacodynamic characteristics of VPA may also affect the relationship between PCOS and VPA. VPA cannot induce the cytochrome P450 enzymes, so it lacks a moderating function for hyperandrogenism, which further increases the risk of PCOS.

In addition to VPA, there are few studies on the effects of traditional antiseizure medications on the reproductive endocrine system of female patients, and research into new antiseizure medications is relatively lagging. At present, no studies have shown that taking the new antiseizure medications such as levetiracetam, oxcarbazepine, perampanel, and lamotrigine will increase the risk of PCOS in WWE. The effects of ASMs on reproductive endocrinology have been attributed in part to the liver enzyme-inducing properties of ASMs. For example, drugs that have liver enzyme-inducing effects include phenytoin and carbamazepine, which can increase SHBG levels and lower testosterone levels. As a result, the hypothalamic-pituitary-ovary axis is affected by negative feedback, GABA, and other mechanisms. However, whether and how most drugs affect reproductive endocrine function through the HPO axis remains to be further studied and determined.

4.2.2 Diagnosis and Treatment of Epilepsy with Comorbid PCOS

4.2.2.1 Diagnosis and Treatment Recommendations of PCOS with Epilepsy

PCOS, as a chronic endocrine and metabolic disease, starts in adolescence and affects women throughout their lives. Although it is difficult to cure it, it can be effectively controlled. Symptomatic treatment should be carried out according to the woman's specific physiological stage to improve their quality of life, and long-term complication prevention and long-term management is required. Individualized comprehensive treatment should be advocated.

1. Lifestyle interventions: Domestic and foreign guidelines advocate that lifestyle intervention is the basic treatment for all patients; that is, comprehensive therapy including balanced diet, reasonable exercise, and behavioral interventions. Comprehensive treatment can not only improve the diet and lifestyle habits of patients, the body's glucose and lipid metabolism, and the body's endocrine state, but also supplement trace elements, promote metabolism, enhance immunity, reduce as well as maintain body weight, and improve the quality of life of patients. Behavioral intervention is an important part of comprehensive treatment, including goal setting, self-monitoring, stimulation control, problem solving improvement, continuous assessment and monitoring, and self-confidence building, in order to optimize body quality management, maintain a healthy lifestyle, and maintain good mood.
2. Adjustment of menstrual cycle: mainly for menstrual disorders and spontaneous menstrual cycles greater than 2 months in patients with no fertility requirements, endometrial long-term pure estrogen stimulation. Approximately 30% of patients with PCOS have endometrial hyperplasia, and the incidence of endometrial cancer is 3–10 times higher than that of the normal population. Depending on different physiological stages and sex hormone levels in the body, periodic progesterone therapy, short-acting combined oral contraceptives (COC), and sequential estrogen progesterone cycle therapy may be considered. Oral contraceptives do not appear to increase the risk of diabetes, but may adversely affect insulin sensitivity and are dose-dependent, and there is insufficient evidence to suggest an increased risk of cardiovascular events in patients with PCOS. However, caution should be used if patients have co-existing risk factors such as hypertension, obesity, blood clotting disorders, and smoking history. The American College of Obstetricians and Gynecologists guidelines state that progesterone therapy alone

or progestogen-containing IUDs are alternatives to endometrial protection, but abnormal uterine bleeding has been reported in 50–89% of patients.

3. Hyperandrogen therapy: short-acting COCs contain estrogen and progesterone and can inhibit hypothalamic-pituitary luteinizing hormone secretion and then inhibit the production of androgens in follicular membrane cells. Estrogen components increase SHBG levels, reduce circulating free testosterone, progesterone can compete to inhibit P450c17/17–20 lyase activity, reduce adrenal androgen production, compete with androgen receptors at the target organ level, and block the peripheral effect of androgen. Long-term use may be effective for hirsute and acne, but may only take effect after 3–6 months. Spironolactone is an antagonistic aldosterone diuretic, which also has the effect of inhibiting ovarian and adrenal anabolic steroids. It can compete with dihydrotestosterone and bind androgen receptors to play an antagonistic androgen effect, and improve the clinical manifestations of hyperandrogenemia, but it may take 6 months or longer to be significantly effective. During the application, one should be alert to potential side effects such as postural hypotension. The use of large doses requires regular monitoring of blood potassium levels.
4. Metabolic disorder adjustment: metformin is an insulin sensitizer that can inhibit intestinal glucose absorption, liver gluconeogenesis and output, increase the uptake and utilization of glucose by tissues, improve insulin sensitivity, and reduce hyperglycemia, but it does not reduce normal blood sugar levels. Pioglitazone is a thiazolidinedione insulin sensitizer that can not only improve insulin sensitivity, but also improve blood lipid metabolism, is anti-inflammatory, and protects the function of vascular endothelial cells. When combined with metformin, it has a synergistic therapeutic effect. Pioglitazone is often used as a combination drug of choice when the efficacy of biguanides is not good, and it is often used in patients with no fertility requirements. Acarbose is a new oral hypoglycemic agent that competitively inhibits glucoside hydrolase in the gut. It reduces the decomposition of polysaccharide and sucrose into glucose, slows down the absorption of sugar accordingly, and reduces postprandial blood sugar. It is generally used alone or in combination with other oral hypoglycemic agents or insulin mellitus.
5. Fertility promotion strategies:
   (a) Pre-pregnancy consultation: Before fertility promotion treatment for infertility patients with PCOS, both couples should be examined to confirm and try to correct the risk factors that may cause fertility failure, such as obesity, uncontrolled glucose tolerance, diabetes, and hypertension. Specific measures include reducing body mass, quitting smoking and alcohol consumption, and controlling blood sugar and blood pressure. Weight reduction is the basic treatment for obese PCOS infertility patients in order to promote fertility. In patients who still do not ovulate after the improvement of metabolic and health problems, drugs can be given to promote ovulation.
   (b) Induction of ovulation: This option is suitable for PCOS patients who have fertility requirements but persistent anovulation or thin ovulation. Other causes of infertility and diseases that are not suitable for pregnancy should

be ruled out before medication. (1) contraceptive: The traditional first-line drug for ovulation induction with PCOS. Starting from the second to fifth day of natural menstruation or withdrawal bleeding, 50 mg/day for a total of 5 days. If there is no ovulation, increase by 50 mg per cycle until reaching 150 mg/day. If the follicular phase is long or the luteal phase is short, the dose may be too low, and the dose can be increased appropriately; if the ovarian stimulation is too large, the dose can be reduced to 25 mg/day. CC alone is recommended for no more than six cycles. (2) letrozole: this can be used as the first-line drug for ovulation induction of PCOS, and can be used for the treatment of patients with CC resistance or failure. From the second to fifth day of natural menstruation or withdrawal bleeding, 2.5 mg/day can be administered for a total of 5 days. If no ovulation occurs, this can be increased by 2.5 mg per cycle until reaching 5.0–7.5 mg/day. (3) Gonadotropins: Commonly used gonadotropins include human menopausal gonadotropin (hMG), high-purity FSH (HP-FSH), and gene recombination FSH (rFSH). It can be used as a combination with CC or letrozole and can also be used as second-line treatment. It may be used in patients with CC resistance and/or failure due to anovulatory infertility.

(c) Laparoscopic ovarian drilling (LOD): this is not commonly recommended and is mainly applicable to patients with CC resistance, ineffective letrozole treatment, refractory excessive LH secretion, laparoscopic pelvic inspection due to other diseases, and inadequate follow-up conditions for gonadotropin therapy monitoring.

(d) In vitro fertilization-embryo transfer (IVF-ET): this is a third-line treatment for infertile patients with PCOS. When PCOS patients have failed the above treatment or when other infertility factors (such as old age, tubal factors, or male factors) are combined, IVF treatment is required. (1) Controlled ovarian hyperstimulation (COH) regimens: PCOS confers high risk for ovarian hyperstimulation syndrome (OHSS), and conventional regimens are not preferred. (2) Whole embryo freezing strategy: this can effectively avoid late-onset OHSS, which is aggravated or induced by endogenous hCG after pregnancy with fresh embryo transfer.

(e) In vitro maturation culture: The application of immature oocyte maturation (IVM) technology in the assisted reproductive treatment of PCOS patients is still controversial. The main indications of IVM in the assisted reproductive treatment of PCOS patients are: (1) insensitivity to ovulation promoting drugs, such as resistance to CC and long-term failure to respond to low dose of gonadotropin, leading to prolonged follicle development or growth; and (2) patients who have experienced moderate to severe OHSS in the past under conventional low-dose gonadotropins.

(f) Application of insulin sensitizers in assisted reproductive therapy: metformin is recommended in the course of assisted reproductive therapy for PCOS patients. Currently, metformin in the treatment of PCOS programs are: (1) alone application: suitable for non-obese PCOS patients (BMI <30 kg/m^2); (2) in combination with CC: for obese PCOS patients; (3)

combined with gonadotropin (hMG or rFSH); and (4) combined with CC or gonadotropin: suitable for patients with CC resistance.

6. Long-term complications and psychological management: Patients' external clinical manifestations, hormone abnormalities, reproductive needs and health problems significantly affect their mental health and quality of life, and studies have shown that psychological disorders are related to being obese/overweight, infertile, and having anxiety and depression. Psychological states can be significantly improved with lifestyle interventions and drug treatment. Conversely, long-term chronic stress exposure can also affect the PCOS phenotype and promote the progression of diseases and complications, including obesity, metabolic disorders, and infertility. Adolescent females have unique social psychological characteristics and are more prone to negative mental health abnormalities. More attention should be paid to adolescent females, and active treatment should be provided if necessary.

There is currently no specific guideline or experts' opinions for the treatment of PCOS in women with epilepsy. Therefore, women who have comorbid epilepsy and PCOS also receive the same standardized PCOS therapy. A symptom-oriented and individualized treatment should be applied in all PCOS patients. As PCOS is a lifelong disorder, practitioners should fully consider patients' needs at different times of their life to achieve successful long-term management. For clinical hyperandrogenism, drugs are not recommended to women seeking fertility. Effective drugs targeting hyperandrogenism include eflornithine for facial hirsutism, retinoids and antibiotics for acne and alopecia, and other anti-androgens such as androgen receptor blockers and 5α-reductase inhibitors. For obesity prevention and management, lifestyle interventions including changes in diet and/or physical activity are recommended for every woman with PCOS. Anti-obesity drugs still lack data about long-term effectiveness. Another option is bariatric surgery. A meta-analysis suggested that bariatric surgery is effective in decreasing serum testosterone levels and relieving hirsutism and menstrual dysfunction. For insulin resistance, metformin is the most used insulin sensitizer drug. And several recommendations support the use of metformin and other sensitizers (thiazolidinediones, berberine, and inositols) in patients with abnormalities in glucose tolerance. For oligo-ovulation, it is important to give individualized treatment considering the patient's desire for fertility. Patients should be referred for assisted reproductive technology when expressing a desire for fertility. For women not seeking fertility, oral contraceptive pills, cyclic or continuous progestin, or levonorgestrel-releasing intrauterine devices could be considered for the prevention of endometrial hyperplasia.

4.2.2.2 Traditional Chinese Medicine Diagnosis and Treatment of Epileptic Comorbidity PCOS

Studies have shown that epilepsy itself may affect the reproductive endocrine function of women, and PCOS has a high incidence even in women with epilepsy who do not take ASMs. However, long-term use of ASMs such as valproic acid can also induce a variety of changes in endocrine function and increase the incidence of epilepsy-related PCOS. Studies have shown that the incidence of epilepsy PCOS in women of childbearing age can reach 26%, more than 1/4 of women with epilepsy are affected by this, and cause reproductive system disorders in women of childbearing age. The main clinical manifestations are menstrual disorders, infertility, postpartum abortion, obesity, hirsutism, and acne.

In view of the limitations of the understanding of the root causes of polycystic ovary syndrome, the current clinical western medicine treatment is the management of specific symptoms. The main treatment methods include adjusting anti-androgen therapy and improving insulin resistance therapy. For women of childbearing age with fertility needs, ovulation induction therapy is essential. Therefore, for female epilepsy patients with PCOS, the clinical medication is complicated and changeable, and they all need to take drugs for a long time to improve their symptoms. However, the long-term use of these drugs can aggravate the occurrence of cardiovascular system, digestive system, and endocrine system diseases, thus facing many challenges in the clinical treatment of PCOS. Traditional Chinese medicine has a long history of understanding of epilepsy and polycystic ovary syndrome and has a unique dialectical thinking and diagnosis and treatment system. In particular, the theoretical guidance of "same treatment for different diseases" in traditional Chinese medicine provides a new idea for the clinical treatment of epilepsy with PCOS.

PCOS primarily results from the malfunctioning of internal organs, characterized by the presence of phlegm and blood stasis. Therefore, the clinical symptoms often manifest as a combination of deficiency and excess, with deficiency as the primary cause and excess as a secondary factor. The onset of the disease is closely associated with the kidneys, spleen, and liver, with kidney and spleen deficiencies being the main contributing factors. Moreover, pathogenic products such as phlegm-dampness and blood stasis impact the body, leading to dysfunction in the "kidney-Tiangui-Chongren-uterine" reproductive axis. Based on various types of syndrome differentiation, PCOS can be categorized into several types: kidney deficiency with excessive phlegm, kidney deficiency with blood stasis, simple kidney deficiency or kidney deficiency mixed with blood stasis and phlegm obstruction, kidney deficiency along with liver and gallbladder heat congestion, elevated liver fire, excessive phlegm, deficiency of spleen and kidney Yang accompanied by phlegm, and spleen and kidney Yin deficiency coupled with emotional depression. The TCM treatment of PCOS is based on the holistic concept and the guidance of syndrome differentiation and treatment theory. In the case of determining the syndrome type of the patient, prescription and medication are used to harmonize the body's qi and blood, restore normal menstruation, and make the ovum develop normally and discharge. At present, there are Chinese medicine sequential therapy, acupuncture, and other treatment methods, which have achieved good clinical curative effect.

Recent studies have shown that seizures may be accompanied by increased pituitary hormone secretion, increased plasma prolactin secretion in patients with complex partial seizures and generalized seizures, and a transient increase in gonadotropins. Studies have shown that epileptic discharges from the amygdala to the hippocampus may stimulate the secretion of gonadotropin-releasing hormone (GnRH), increase the frequency of GnRH pulses, promote the secretion of LH, inhibit the secretion of FSH, and increase the LH/FSH ratio. The left temporal lobe has a higher LH pulse frequency than the right temporal lobe, so patients with left temporal lobe-marginal lobe epileptic discharges are prone to PCOS; on the contrary, anovulatory cycles can induce epileptiform discharges in the limbic lobe, and progesterone can increase the threshold of epileptic seizures. In women with anovulatory epilepsy, including PCOS, progesterone levels are reduced. In addition, the temporal lobe-marginal lobe structure of anovulatory women is sensitive to estrogen, which can lead to secondary seizures. Patients with epilepsy and reproductive endocrine disorders often have neurotransmission dysfunction or genetic defects, indicating that they play a role in the relationship between PCOS and epilepsy.

TCM treatment: TCM treatment of PCOS focuses on the etiology and pathogenesis, such as kidney deficiency and blood stasis syndrome patients, the treatment to promote blood stasis, tonifying liver and kidney, tonifying Qi and spleen, and nourishing Chongren, can be used to promote follicle development, such as Guiliongdihuang Decoction, Yishen Huoxue Xiaoshi decoction. The treatment principle of patients with phlegm-dampness internal obstruction syndrome is to remove phlegm and remove dampness, Kujiangxin, eliminating ruffian and dispersing. Banxia Xiexin Decoction and Cangfu Daotan Decoction can be used to alleviate disease symptoms, regulate metabolic indexes, and improve reproductive health. Patients with kidney deficiency and liver depression syndrome can tonify kidney and regulate liver, promote Qi and blood, make liver Qi reach, Chongren Tongsheng, it is easier to conceive, commonly used prescriptions are polycystic drink, Danggui Shaoyao powder and so on.

Acupuncture and moxibustion treatment: Acupuncture and moxibustion is a traditional Chinese medicine therapy, the mechanism of the treatment of PCOS is carried out from many aspects. Acupuncture has a stimulating effect on the hypothalamic-pituitary-gonadal axis and can improve the low sex hormone state. At the same time, acupuncture can regulate the production of central β-endorphin, which is closely related to the functional regulation of the hypothalamic-pituitary-gonadal axis, regulate the rhythm of β-endorphin secretion, and can regulate the level of hypothalamic gonadotropin-releasing hormone. Secondly, acupuncture also acts on the hypothalamic-pituitary-adrenal axis, which can promote the release of adrenocorticotropin, improve the level of estrogen, and indirectly affect the secretion of pituitary hormones. In addition, acupuncture and moxibustion also has a certain impact on the endocrine and metabolic system, which can improve insulin resistance and reduce insulin levels, so as to achieve the effect of reducing gonadotropin and androgen levels and increasing follicle stimulating hormone levels.

Auricular point sticking: According to the meridians theory of traditional Chinese medicine, auricular point is closely related to various organs and tissues of the human body. Auricle sticking treatment uses medical tape to precisely stick the drug seeds to the corresponding acupuncture points in the ear, with manual pressure, so that patients feel sour, numbness, and swelling pain, so as to play the therapeutic effect. Commonly used medicine seeds are white mustard seeds, Wang do not line seeds, Zhongcheng pills, etc. Wang do not line seeds are used more because of hard material and good efficacy. By continuously stimulating the corresponding acupoints for a long time, the zang-fu organs can be adjusted to Chongren, Qi-blood operation, and the ovarian function of patients can be effectively regulated.

For patients with epilepsy and PCOS, while effectively controlling seizures, it can also effectively promote follicular development, promote ovulation, improve endometrial receptivity, regulate lipid metabolism, and reduce insulin resistance, thereby improving PCOS symptoms such as oligomenorrhea, infertility, and obesity.

4.3 Pre-pregnancy Counseling for Women with Epilepsy

Ziyi Chen

4.3.1 Counseling for Pregnancy Preparation

Female patients with epilepsy should conduct routine pre-pregnancy consultation before pregnancy, and choose the best time to conceive through pre-pregnancy assessment, in order to reduce the risk of fetal abnormalities and children's intellectual development disorders. Women of childbearing age should consult epilepsy specialists and obstetricians before they have the intention to become pregnant. The doctor should explain how seizures themselves and ASMs affect a woman's fertility, and inform her of seizure-related obstetric complications. If there is a family history of epilepsy or if hereditary epilepsy is suspected, it is recommended to consult a geneticist for genetic counseling before making pregnancy decisions.

4.3.1.1 Pre-pregnancy Medication Management

Long-term ASM use will have an impact on female hormones; for example, long-term use of valproic acid may increase the risk of hyperandrogenemia and polycystic ovary syndrome and can even affect fertility. In addition, the long-term use of ASMs has varying degrees of impact on maternal and offspring, will increase the occurrence of pregnancy complications and adverse outcomes of offspring, and previous studies have shown that the risk of ASMs teratogenesis is related to the type of drug, dose level, and whether a multi-drug treatment approach was used. Therefore, for WWE of childbearing age who have fertility needs, medication management should be optimized from the pre-pregnancy preparation stages.

If a patient has not had seizures in the preceding 3–5 years and their EEG is normal, one can consider phasing out the drug by referring to the general principles for ASM reduction. However, one should fully inform the patient in advance of the possible recurrence of epilepsy and its impact on the patient and the fetus. If a patient cannot reach the goal of drug reduction and still need to take long-term medication, there should be a comprehensive assessment of the condition, and according to the type of seizures of patients, choose the minimum dose ASMs required to control seizures, with a preference for some new ASMs (recommended levetiracetam, oxcarbazepine, and lamotrigine). As far as possible, the use of valproic acid should be avoided and monotherapy is also recommended. It is worth noting that, relative to other ASMs, valproic acid as a single or combined drug, especially when the total dose is >1000 mg/day, is associated with an increased risk of the fetus suffering from neural tube defects, spina bifida, and genitourinary system congenital malformations. Therefore, for patients who take this type of ASM, even if it is suitable for the patient's epilepsy type, it should be recommended that the clinician re-evaluate and choose alternative ASMs before the woman considers pregnancy. In addition, prior to changing medications, one should ensure that an effective blood concentration is achieved prior to pregnancy. For women who are on combination therapy, it is not clinically recommended to stop taking medications completely before becoming pregnant, given the short golden age for women to have children and the low teratogenic risk associated with most low-dose ASMs. Instead, ASM use should be adjusted according to the patient's specific situation: a. Change to low-dose monotherapy; b. Substitute drugs with high teratogenic rates; and c. Maintain the original regimen but reduce the dose.

ASMs are prescribed to reduce the severity of epilepsy during pregnancy, however, the adverse reactions of ASMs on the fetus of WWE cannot be ignored. The effects of ASMs on embryos or fetuses are mainly manifested in the following three aspects: (1) major congenital malformations (MCMs); (2) neurodevelopmental disorders; and (3) fetal growth restriction. Current studies consistently show that second-generation ASMs such as LTG and LEV are significantly superior to traditional ASMs such as VPA, CBZ, and PHT in terms of drug safety, teratogenicity, and impact on the neurodevelopment of offspring. Tomson T. et al. classified the teratogenic risk of ASMs with reasonable data: low risk, including LTG, LEV, OXC, CBZ, and GBP; PB, TPM, and PHT as medium risk; and VPA as high risk. As for type of malformations, cardiac malformations are the most common major congenital malformations after exposed to ASMs in uterine, while others include neural tube defects, cleft lip and palate, hypospadias, and skeletal malformations. Therefore, it is recommended that safer ASMs such as LTG or LEV should be used whenever possible in pregnancy WWE for the health of offspring.

4.3.1.2 Degree of Pre-pregnancy Epilepsy Control

The seizures themselves will also affect WWE hormone levels and, in turn, WWE fertility. Preconception seizure-free time is associated with the degree of seizure control during pregnancy. Studies from European and Australian epileptic pregnancy registries have shown that the duration of preconception seizure-free duration is an important predictor of seizures during pregnancy. Women with seizure-free intervals 9–12 months before pregnancy have an 82–94% chance of remaining seizure-free during pregnancy. In addition, there is more evidence that poor seizure control during pregnancy has adverse effects on the mother and the fetus itself, and the occurrence of comprehensive tonic-clonic seizures during pregnancy is easy to cause stillbirth, abortion, and other adverse pregnancy outcomes, which is also one of the main causes of accidental death in women with epilepsy patients. Other, less severe seizures that damage the state of consciousness also carry a greater risk for pregnant women and fetuses. Therefore, in order to achieve a seizure-free pregnancy, in addition to the standardized management of pregnancy, pre-pregnancy seizure control management is also our focus. However, at present, there is no international consensus opinion on preconception seizure-free time, and according to the existing women with epilepsy management guidelines we recommend that women with epilepsy of childbearing age attain at least 9 months of seizure freedom before planning pregnancy.

4.3.1.3 Other Management Before Pregnancy

Low levels of folic acid are associated with neural tube defects, abortion, and intrauterine fetal growth inhibition. Daily supplementation of small doses of folic acid plays an important role in the prevention of neural tube malformations. The NEAD study also showed that folic acid supplementation in women with epilepsy was beneficial for the psychomotor development of the fetus after birth. It is generally believed that women with epilepsy who take ASMs need to supplement more folic acid than the general population, especially when preparing for pregnancy and when taking ASMs that are antagonists of folic acid, such as valproic acid, phenobarbital, phenytoin, and carbamazepine. However, there is currently no consensus on the recommended dosage of folic acid supplementation. China's recommendations on folic acid supplementation are as follows: women with epilepsy should take folic acid supplements every day from the time of conception, and continue until at least 12 weeks of pregnancy. If a woman is not taking ASMs, the recommended daily dose of folic acid is 0.4 mg; if she is taking folic acid antagonists, has a history of miscarriage, or has produced a neural tube teratoma, the recommended daily dose of folic acid is 5 mg.

In addition, in order to facilitate adjustment of the dose according to the blood concentration during pregnancy, it is recommended to monitor the blood concentration of ASMs before pregnancy as the baseline reference for the adjustment of the blood concentration during pregnancy. The fertility of WWE is lower than that of non-women with epilepsy, so in order to improve fertility, in addition to the pre-pregnancy preparation of WWE themselves, it is recommended to check the sperm of the pre-pregnancy spouse to prevent the failure of planned pregnancy or possible problems of the spouse.

4.3.2 Genetic Counseling

The 2014 Epilepsy Cause Classification study showed that most epilepsy is genetically related. Most of the genes involved in epilepsy are expressed in the brain and code for ion channel subunits that stabilize and transmit neural activity. When these genes are mutated in a pathogenic way, they lead to seizures. Clinical hereditary epilepsy includes two categories, one is epilepsy as the only or main clinical symptoms of the syndrome, that is, idiopathic epilepsy, where an increasing number of pathogenic genes have been reported. The other is inherited metabolic diseases, chromosomal diseases, mitochondrial genetic diseases combined with epilepsy, where epilepsy is one of the symptoms of brain damage. Idiopathic epileptic syndromes with known pathogenic genes include benign familial neonatal convulsions, benign familial infantile convulsions, absence epilepsy in children, absence epilepsy in adolescents, idiopathic generalized epilepsy, juvenile myoclonic epilepsy, benign adult familial myoclonic epilepsy, general epilepsy with paroxysmal dyskinesia, febrile convulsions combined with general epileptic adjunctive disorder, and infantile myoclonus gravis epilepsy, benign childhood epilepsy with centrotemporal spines, autosomal dominant nocturnal frontal lobe epilepsy, and familial temporal lobe epilepsy. Clinical features, electrophysiological manifestations, and family history need to be defined for this type of epileptic syndrome. Mitochondrial genetic disorders associated with epilepsy include Unverricht-Lundborg progressive myoclonic epilepsy and Lafora progressive myoclonic epilepsy. Genetic metabolic diseases associated with epilepsy include Gaucher's disease type III, sialidosis, neuronal ceroid lipofuscinoses storage disease, pyridoxal deficiency, Down syndrome, Angelman syndrome, Fragile X syndrome, and tuberous sclerosis. Attention should be paid to other signs and symptoms of the nervous system, special features and body types, manifestations of damage to other systems, and family history of these genetic disorders.

Patients with epilepsy should be evaluated for genetic risk prior to pregnancy, and there are currently no guidelines to recommend routine pre-pregnancy genetic testing for women with epilepsy. Patients need to be consulted before pregnancy by epilepsy specialists to understand their medical history in detail, in addition to the patient's clinical information, electroencephalogram, imaging, other auxiliary examination results, and further detail on the patient's family history. According to the above data evaluation, it should be judged whether the patient has a hereditary epilepsy syndrome. In the case of non-hereditary epilepsy, the offspring have only a slightly increased susceptibility to epilepsy without additional intervention. If the possibility of inheritance is considered, the patient needs to undergo genetic testing and, if inherited epilepsy is confirmed, they need to be referred to the fetal medical center to undergo disease-causing gene screening. Some patients can consider IVF.

References

Herzog AG, Mandle HB, Cahill KE, et al. Contraceptive practices of women with epilepsy: findings of the epilepsy birth control registry. Epilepsia. 2016;57(4):630–7.

Lai W, et al. Plasma luteinizing hormone level affects the brain activity of patients with polycystic ovary syndrome. Psychoneuroendocrinology. 2020;112:104535.

Reddy DS. Do oral contraceptives increase epileptic seizures? Expert Rev Neurother. 2017;17(2):129–34.

Verrotti A, D'Egidio C, Mohn A, Coppola G, Parisi P, Chiarelli F. Antiepileptic drugs, sex hormones, and PCOS. Epilepsia. 2011;52(2):199–211.

Suggested Readings

Escobar-Morreale HF. Polycystic ovary syndrome: definition, aetiology, diagnosis and treatment. Nat Rev Endocrinol. 2018;14(5):270–84.

Goodarzi MO, Dumesic DA, Chazenbalk G, et al. Polycystic ovary syndrome: etiology, pathogenesis and diagnosis. Nat Rev Endocrinol. 2011;7(4):219–31.

Gooneratne IK, Wimalaratna M, Ranaweera AKP, et al. Contraception advice for women with epilepsy. BMJ. 2017;357:j2010.

Guo J, Liu Y, Kong L, et al. Comparison of the probability of four anticonvulsant mood stabilizers to facilitate polycystic ovary syndrome in women with epilepsies or bipolar disorder—a systematic review and meta-analysis. Front Psych. 2023;14:1128011.

Halane HIM, Hargreave M, Kjaer SK, et al. Maternal use of hormonal contraception and epilepsy in offspring. Hum Reprod. 2021;36(6):1674–81.

Herzog AG. Catamenial epilepsy: definition, prevalence pathophysiology and treatment. Seizure. 2008;17(2):151–9.

Herzog AG, Mandle HB, Maceachern DB. Prevalence of highly effective contraception use by women with epilepsy. Neurology. 2019;92(24):e2815–21.

Huang S. Research progress on the etiology and treatment of polycystic ovary syndrome in traditional Chinese and Western medicine. Electron J Mod Med Health Res. 2023;7(11):130–3.

Huang H, Hu X, Xu M. Contraceptive management of women with epilepsy in childbearing age. J Clin Neurol. 2019;32(02):146–9.

King A, Gerard EE. Contraception, fecundity, and pregnancy in women with epilepsy: an update on recent literature. Curr Opin Neurol. 2022;35(2):161–8.

Kirkpatrick L, Van Cott AC, Kazmerski TM, et al. Contraception and reproductive health care for adolescent and young adult women with epilepsy. J Pediatr. 2022;241:229–36.

Li S, Zhang L, Wei N, et al. Research progress on the effect of epilepsy and antiseizure medications on PCOS through HPO axis. Front Endocrinol (Lausanne). 2021;12:787854.

Markoula S, et al. Reproductive health in patients with epilepsy. Epilepsy Behav. 2020;113:107563.

Mccartney CR, Marshall JC. Clinical practice. Polycystic ovary syndrome. N Engl J Med. 2016;375(1):54–64.

Song Y, Li R. Interpretation of the Chinese diagnosis and treatment guidelines for polycystic ovary syndrome. Pract J Obstet Gynecol. 2018;34(10):737–41.

Sun W, Wang W, Wu X. Epilepsy, antiepileptic drugs and polycystic ovary syndrome in women. Chin J Rehabil Theory Pract. 2006;03:232–4.

Zhou JQ, Zhou LM, Chen LJ, et al. Polycystic ovary syndrome in patients with epilepsy: a study in 102 Chinese women. Seizure. 2012;21(9):729–7.

Perinatal Management of Women with Epilepsy

5

Ziyi Chen, Zhenlei Wang, Sijia Basang, and Leihao Sha

5.1 Management of Epilepsy During Pregnancy

Ziyi Chen

Seizures during pregnancy will have adverse effects on the mother and fetus, so in addition to routine prenatal examination, female patients during pregnancy should also visit the epilepsy specialist regularly to dynamically assess whether they still have seizures and to determine the type of seizures, in order to adjust the dose and type of drugs in a timely fashion.

In the prepregnancy assessment, if one cannot reduce the ASMs of WWE, the patient should adhere to medication during pregnancy so as to avoid the recurrence of seizure activity and its related adverse consequences. Previous studies have shown that the occurrence of tonic-clonic seizures during pregnancy will not only cause an increased risk of epileptic falls and blunt trauma in WWE, but also increases the risk of hypoxemia and asphyxia to the fetus, as well as fetal bradycardia, hypoxia, stillbirth, and abortion, and can also cause accidental death in pregnant women with epilepsy. Although focal seizures during pregnancy are considered unlikely to have a significant impact on the fetus, there is also evidence that they may lead to transient fetal distress and slowed fetal heart rate. Poor seizure control

Z. Chen
Department of Neurology, The First Affiliated Hospital, Sun Yat-sen University, Guangzhou, China
e-mail: chenziyi@mail.sysu.edu.cn

Z. Wang (✉)
Clinical Trial Center, West China Hospital, Sichuan University, Chengdu, China
e-mail: wangzhenlei@wchscu.cn

S. Basang · L. Sha
Department of Neurology, West China Hospital, Sichuan University, Chengdu, China

L. Chen (ed.), *Women with Epilepsy in Child-bearing Age*,
https://doi.org/10.1007/978-981-97-3921-9_5

during pregnancy should be considered in addition to the possible association with severe vomiting in the first trimester and decreased blood concentration during pregnancy. Compliance with WWE medication during pregnancy should also be a key concern. Random discontinuation of medication during pregnancy can lead to recurrent seizures during pregnancy and worsening of the severity and frequency of seizures during pregnancy, which is harmful to the mother and the fetus.

Clinical Recommendations for Management of Epilepsy During Pregnancy
Currently, the ASMs used in clinical practice can almost pass the placental barrier; thus, considering the potential adverse effects of ASMs on pregnancy outcomes, WWE should be careful when taking drugs and should consult epilepsy specialists before pregnancy for pregnancy medication adjustment. The goal during pregnancy is, as far as reasonably practical, to use the lowest dose of recognized pregnancy-safe monotherapy ASM. We recommend that all ASM adjustments are completed before conception, and that the use of traditional ASMs such as valproic acid, phenytoin, and phenobarbital should be avoided as much as possible during pregnancy. However, for patients who still use VPA for different reasons before pregnancy and for unplanned pregnancies, temporary replacement of VPA during pregnancy is not recommended if the seizures are well controlled, and adjustment to a lower dose can be achieved. If epilepsy is not well controlled, one can try to switch to one of the new ASMs (such as zonisamide and lacosamide) with a faster onset under the guidance of a professional doctor, or add a new ASM while maintaining a lower VPA dose.

5.2 Monitoring and Early Warning of Seizures

Sijia Basang

Epilepsy is one of the commonest chronic neurological disorders worldwide, affecting more than 70 million patients globally. Due to the unpredictability of epileptic seizures, patients with sudden disturbance of consciousness during epileptic seizures may suffer accidental injuries such as falls, burns, drowning, and traffic accidents. The risk of sudden accidental death in patients with epilepsy is 27 times that of sudden death in the general population, second only to stroke among neurological diseases. The unpredictability and uncertainty of seizures is distressing for patients and caregivers, affecting their quality of life, employability, and even life safety. In order to reduce the serious disease burden caused by seizures, artificial intelligence (AI), wearable devices (WDs), and implantable devices have been developed in recent years. With the deepening of research into the mechanisms of epilepsy and the discovery of new biomarkers, the study of seizure monitoring and early warnings based on various indicators has become a hot spot and focus in the epilepsy research field. Epilepsy monitoring and early warning offers the possibility to warn patients so that they can divert or initiate interventions in a timely manner, such as acute, fast-acting drugs or implantable controls, and provide seizure data to the medical team to reduce response times to the patient. Table 5.1 summarized the seizure monitoring and early warning equipment from previous literatures.

5.2.1 Electroencephalogram

Electroencephalogram (EEG) analysis is widely used in neuroscience, especially in the diagnosis and monitoring of epilepsy. High-precision automated seizure detection systems will simplify clinical practice and speed up intervention or preventive treatment for patients at risk of seizures. In recent years, with the gradual development of precision medicine, a large number of studies have proved that the automatic recognition and detection of epileptic seizures on EEG based on various algorithms makes accurate seizure monitoring and prediction possible. Currently, most studies have classified brain states between and before seizures based on intracranial EEG (iEEG) and scalp EEG (sEEG) processing characteristics, resulting in a number of excellent algorithm models. The algorithms usually follow the same basic scheme: (1) acquisition and preprocessing of EEG; (2) extraction of EEG features, with commonly used feature extraction analysis methods including linear dynamic analysis (time domain, frequency domain, and time–frequency domain), nonlinear dynamic analysis, and brain network analysis; and (3) classification recognition of EEG, with the extracted features used in decision algorithms for modeling and classification in order to monitor or predict seizures.

Public databases are the source of data for most current seizure monitoring and prediction research. In 2013, the world's first human clinical trial in the field demonstrated the feasibility of prospective seizure prediction in long-term iEEG records, overcoming the limitations of short recording time and limited number of seizure events in traditional EEG data (Cook et al. 2013). The EPILEPSIAE database, the most comprehensive epilepsy database available, is fully annotated by EEG experts and contains high-quality long-term EEG recordings, derived features, clinical information, and imaging data. In addition, databases such as IEEG.org, CHB-MIT, and others are also included. However, the use of databases means that most of the current studies lack effective prospective validation (Sahu et al. 2020; Gabeff et al. 2021; Reuben et al. 2020).

A reasonable and effective feature extraction method is a prerequisite and key to the successful construction of the model. Since the 1980s, people have used time and frequency domain analysis to predict epileptic seizures. However, the waveform of time domain analysis is susceptible to interference, the data representation is poor, and frequency domain analysis cannot provide good temporal resolution. In order to overcome these limitations, various time–frequency domain analysis methods are proposed, which not only provide joint distribution information of time domain and frequency domain, but also clearly describe the relationship between signal frequency and time change. Later, a large number of published studies confirmed that nonlinear analysis can accurately identify the dynamic changes before epileptic seizures, thus predicting epileptic seizures. Commonly used features include correlation dimension, correlation entropy, noise level, Lempel-Ziv

Table 5.1 Seizure monitoring and early warning equipment

Device name	Device form	Signal acquisition	Algorithm	Effectiveness	interactivity	Other functions
NextSense	Earplug	Ear-EEG ACC ECG	SVM	SS = 84–100% FAR = 5/24–13/24 h	Digital platform	Cognitive assessment, self-reporting, performance monitoring, drug tracking, privacy protection
RNS system	Implantable brain stimulation devices (chip implants)	EEG	GLM	Training set: IoC = 15/18 Validation set: IoC = 104/157	–	Delivers precise electrical stimulation to the patient's brain to suppress seizures
Empatica E4	Wrist strap	EDA, ACC, BVP, TEMP, HR	LSTM	IoC = 28.5% SS = 75.6% TiW = 47.2	Alert App Mate App Empatica	Seizure diary, medication reminder, data visualization, analysis rest
None	Bipolar leads	HRV	MSPC	SS = 85.7% FAR = 0.62/h	Smart phone	–
Truenorth	Chip	EEG	DL	SS = 69% TIW = 27%	–	–
EDDI	Attach to the bicep	sEMG	–	SS = 93.8% FAR = 0.67/d	Computer	
Epi-Care	Wrist strap	ACC	–	SS = 90% FAR = 0.1/d	Epi-Care	Call, locate, alert and forward

Nightwatch	Bracelet	HR, ACC	–	SS = 86% FAR = 0.03/	Base station, Macbook Infrared sensitive camera	
None	Electrodes are placed laterally on the biceps	sEMG	GLM	All GTCS detected, FAR =1.4/24 h	Base station computer	–
EMFIT	Bed sensor	Motion (breathing, heart rate)	–	All day ACC = 29.5% Night ACC = 53.6%	–	–

complexity, and maximum Lyapunov index. However, there are changes in the functional connectivity characteristics of the brain network during seizures, so there is a certain amount of missing information in both linear and nonlinear methods. In recent years, seizure prediction methods have increasingly focused on the analysis and modeling of brain networks, emphasizing local and global connectivity, mutuality, and synchronization. Common brain network features include phase correlation, nonlinear partially directed coherence, centrality, and periodic components of the network. In addition, with the development of long-range electrophysiological detection techniques, a large number of studies have confirmed that seizures are co-regulated by cycles running on different timescales, from shorter cycles (<24 h) to longer cycles (1 week–1 year). Therefore, a combined model that adds cycle information can maximize the performance of seizure prediction algorithms, which proves to be one of the most significant breakthroughs in this field in recent years. In the face of complex and diverse EEG data, it is necessary to comprehensively use multiple feature extraction methods to mine multi-dimensional EEG features. Compared with studies based on a single feature, integrating multiple feature types can significantly improve predictive performance.

In recent years, with the development of artificial intelligence technology, machine learning (ML), and deep learning (DL) can objectively and accurately analyze and model large and complex EEG data, and thus quantify the degree of brain anatomical and functional abnormalities caused by epilepsy (Harden et al. 2009). This is helpful for seizure monitoring and prediction. Wearable devices are also expected to overcome various limitations of EEG devices and meet the needs of patients for daily use. We will introduce the application of artificial intelligence algorithms and wearable devices in seizure monitoring and early warning in detail in the following chapters (Mckee et al. 2023).

5.2.2 Artificial Intelligence Monitoring of Seizures

With the development of precision medicine, a large number of studies have proved that the automatic recognition and detection of EEG based on various ML algorithms make accurate seizure monitoring and prediction possible. The problem of automatic detection of epileptic EEG signals can be transformed into the problem of classification of EEG signals. There are two kinds of classification methods. One is to determine whether epilepsy occurs or not based on the kinetic index reaching a set threshold. The other is to label the segmented EEG as preseizure, interseizure, and seizure. Predictions made during the preseizure period are considered true predictions, predictions made outside the preseizure period are considered false predictions, and the best classifier is selected by comparing the performance of different classifiers. A variety of machine learning algorithms have been applied in this area, including support vector machines (SVM), Bayesian linear discriminant analysis (BLDA), decision tree (DT), extreme learning machine (ELM), k-means clustering algorithm, gradient boosting decision tree (GBDT), and logistic regression. Although some traditional machine learning techniques are reasonably accurate, they often require complex feature engineering. In many fields, deep learning has achieved far higher accuracy than classical ML methods, and deep neural network technology is also widely used in the field of seizure monitoring and early warning. Compared with classical ML algorithms, DL does not require feature engineering; it is easy to migrate and can make the pre-trained deep network effective for different applications in the same field through transfer learning. If the amount of data is sufficiently large, the deep network can be better scaled. Compared with ML, DL has obvious advantages in seizure detection, among which convolutional neural networks (CNN) are the most widely used. Artificial and recurrent neural networks are also commonly used DL models. In addition, generative adversarial networks (GANs) trained by unsupervised learning have been applied to seizure prediction based on retroaural EEG, achieving a sensitivity of 96.3%. Since EEG is a highly dynamic and nonlinear time series data in nature, long short-term memory (LSTM) has certain advantages in sequence modeling problems, and it has thus also been applied to seizure prediction in recent years. Tsiouris et al. and Kostas Manas et al. with LSTM, Kostas Manas et al. obtained a sensitivity close to 100% by extracting time domain, frequency domain, mutual correlation, and graph theory features to predict seizures. Compared with CNN, graph convolutional neural networks (GCNNs) treat EEG regions as nodes in the topology and use edges to represent the relationship between them, which can retain richer connection information. The predictive performance of DL is significantly improved, but it usually leads to a black box model lacking interpretability, which is unable to reflect the true association between seizures and features, has low security, and other problems. Therefore, Gao et al. proposed the multiscale prototype partial network, which is the most advanced self-explanatory model in the field of epilepsy prediction. Interpretable models have the following advantages: high transparency, easier to incorporate into clinical practice, important intervention factors can be identified, provision of key clues for causal studies, improved model prediction performance, and the creation of models that conform to ethical and legal needs. Interpretability models may be a key research direction in the field of seizure prediction in the future.

Also, how does one make a good enough prediction? How does one know the generalization power of the model? How does one choose a good model? Algorithmic ecosystems and big international competitions may be the answer to these questions. Epilepsyecosystem.org (https://www.epilepsyecosystem.org) is an ecological system data and algorithm in constant development that is committed to jointly solving the problem of epileptic seizure prediction. The system provides an online environment that uses competition data and the source code of the best-performing algorithms to further improve the algorithms. Developers are able to download high-quality competition data and train the algorithms independently, visualize the data, and access, share, and discuss the code. Algorithm performance is evaluated by independent evaluators, and the top algorithms in the ecosystem participate in full clinical trials. Such evaluations will facilitate identification of the best seizure prediction algorithm for the broadest range of patients and provide a platform for large-scale prospective clinical trials for seizure prediction. Another advantage of the algorithmic ecosystem is that strong learners can be obtained by combining different algorithms in an intelligent way by combining the complementary outputs of the top algorithms through ensemble learning. However, for some patients whose epilepsy is difficult to predict, there may be an upper bound on the predictive performance of epilepsy through machine learning approaches. More targeted approaches need to be considered from multiple perspectives. For example, more in-depth research into preseizure mechanisms, taking into account clinical factors, exploring more variables associated with seizures, targeting patients' sleep-wake rhythms, and utilizing new types of high-quality wearable devices may provide further benefits for these patients (Sahu et al. 2020).

5.2.3 Wearable Seizure Monitoring Devices

Although the use of EEG signals for seizure prediction has achieved reliable sensitivity and specificity, the use of EEG devices in daily life is not practical, EEG devices are expensive, the instrument is cumbersome to operate, and conductive gels need to be applied to the head of the person being tested in order for the device to fit onto the scalp. In addition, subjects are kept motionless for long periods of time, and vEEG monitoring of hospitalized patients fails to capture seizures in up to one-third of patients. As a result, wearable devices are rapidly gaining a foothold in the field of seizure monitoring and prediction due to their powerful interactivity and portability (Lyu et al. 2021).

Invented and developed under the trend of miniaturization and portability of computers and electronic products, wearable devices collect human physiological data through hardware devices and realize cloud interaction of data through software systems to monitor and evaluate users' health conditions, and then provide users with personalized services. With the real-time monitoring and alarm function of wearable devices, patients can relieve the tension and anxiety associated with a disease at any time, so as to improve the quality of life of patients and reduce the risk of SUDEP. On the other hand, such devices can automatically help patients establish epilepsy logs, overcome the problem of missing reports caused by manual records, and provide a basis for doctors to evaluate the condition and formulate the next treatment plan.

Since epilepsy is a chronic disease, the system for acquiring and processing the body's physiological signals should be long-term so that it can be implanted or carried by the patient to provide real-time predictions. Wearable devices, and especially implantable devices, require a low power budget to achieve long-term operation. In addition, reliable monitoring and early warning with high sensitivity and specificity are required to reduce the number of missed alarms and false positives, ensuring the effectiveness of the system and minimal disruption to patients' daily lives. Communication modules should also be in place to automatically send alerts to relatives or caregivers for timely intervention. Real-time epilepsy detection and monitoring integrated with wearable devices and a variety of signals, as well as predictive analysis of biomedical signals based on neural network systems, have the characteristics of short processing time and low computing power, and are essential for early warning and intervention for patients with epilepsy.

The RNS system is a direct brain reactive neural stimulation system. When the EEG captured meets a certain epileptic threshold, the cranial electrical stimulator will send electrical stimulation to the epileptic focus through deep electrodes to suppress the epileptic seizure. Sigge Weisdorf et al. implanted the SubQ system under the skin of nine patients with temporal lobe epilepsy, which proved the device to be feasible, safe, and well tolerated during home monitoring for up to 3 months. Compared with traditional EEG instruments or polysomnography, sleeping with earplugs has less impact on sleep and can be monitored for a long time. NextSense uses earplugs to perform postauricular electroencephalography, and a number of studies have proved that the device can record seizure activity with almost the same accuracy as traditional EEG. However, the performance of retroauricular-based EEG seizure detection devices decreases when few electrodes are used and spatial sampling is reduced, and convincing evidence for the accuracy of these devices is still lacking.

Seizures can lead to changes in the autonomic function of the heart, and the amount of preseizure information contained in a single-channel ECG may be comparable to sEEG with up to 21 channels due to heart rate variability (HRV) in the preseizure phase. Changes in HRV have been reported in association with epilepsy and therefore a number of studies have developed a seizure prediction model based on the time and frequency domain characteristics of HRV, combined with ML algorithms such as SVM, which can give an alarm as early as 30 min before the onset of seizures. However, HRV research is limited by inconsistent experimental protocols, and these studies are often ineffective, hindering clinical practice. In addition, electrodermal activity (EDA) is a measurement of skin conductivity, which reflects the activity of the sympathetic nervous system. It is collected based on WDs and often integrates multimodal physiological information such as acceleration, heart rate, blood pressure, body temperature and oxygen saturation, and is combined with CNN or LSTM algorithms for seizure prediction. However, it currently only has better predictive performance than random. Gregg et al. also proved that the periodic regulation of the above physiological signals is related to seizures, and periodic features such as circadian rhythm and multi-day heart rate cycle provide the possibility of long-term monitoring and can predict the risk of seizures up to 3 days in advance. In general, ECG- and EDA-based seizure prediction has good portability, but there are few effective identifiable features before seizure onset, and the predictive performance is still far behind that of EEG.

Although wearable devices have made rapid progress in seizure prediction and detection in the last 20 years, false alarms pose a challenge to objective quantification of seizures using wearable devices. Due to the lack of quality evaluation and long-term supervision system, the monitoring data is inaccurate and incomparable. At the same time, the lack of data information standards and docking norms seriously restricts the recognition and utilization of wearable device data. In the future, it will be important to focus on improving the quality of evaluation and supervision systems within wearable devices. The development of wearable devices for seizure prediction not only depends on a deeper understanding of the mechanism of epilepsy, but also depends on the development of artificial intelligence, mechanical engineering, and other fields. With the progress of technology and theory, wearable devices in the future will rely on recorded physiological, behavioral, and environmental data to form a service closed-loop. Monitoring data could help doctors more clearly and accurately understand the changes in patients' physical conditions and better develop personalized solutions, so as to improve the quality of medical services provided to patients with epilepsy.

5.2.4 Advances in Monitoring and Early Warning of Seizures

Neuroimaging: The emergence of neuroimaging technology has realized the visualization and quantification of brain structural and functional abnormalities, which has brought an opportunity for seizure monitoring and early warning. At present, the imaging features used to predict seizures are mainly functional, such as functional near-infrared spectroscopy (fNIRS) and resting state functional magnetic resonance imaging. Since the neuronal changes before a seizure can lead to changes in blood oxygen level dependent (BOLD) activity, in 2019, Rosas-Romero et al. used CNN and fNIRS signals for the first time to predict seizures with an accuracy range of 96.9–100%, which is significantly better than conventional EEG. In addition, Hossein et al. developed a multimodal unsupervised seizure prediction model based on EEG and resting state fMRI data combined with SVM and CNN, with an accuracy of 98%. Brain inflammation is an important factor in the transformation of a healthy brain into an "epileptic brain," and imaging of inflammatory biomarker translocation proteins by positron emission tomography can accurately predict the frequency of spontaneous recurrent seizures (SRS). In a recent study, Zhang et al. developed a novel imaging biomarker based on oxygen-glucose index (OGI) metabolism. During the interseizure period, the OGI in the hippocampus of patients with temporal lobe epilepsy was higher than that on the healthy side. However, the validity of these features needs to be further verified, and the image-based approach cannot achieve long-term seizure prediction in daily life.

Molecular biomarkers: At present, there are few studies on molecular biomarkers for seizure prediction. Since inducing seizures may be related to activation of the blood–brain barrier, Bronisz et al. evaluated serum protein levels associated with the blood–brain barrier and found that serum levels of MMP-2, MMP-9, and CCL-2 could be used as potential biomarkers for predicting seizures. Marion et al. conducted small RNA sequencing of plasma samples collected during vEEG monitoring in patients with focal epilepsy and found that three tRNA fragments (5′, 5′ AlaTGC, and 5′ GluCTC) were higher before and after seizures, suggesting that they may serve as biomarkers of seizure risk in patients with epilepsy (AUC = 0.8–0.95) and these potential markers may be used in the future to predict the onset of epilepsy or evaluate the prognosis of epilepsy [68]. Branched chain amino acids (BCAAs) play an important role in glutaminergic neurotransmission, mitochondrial function, neurodegeneration, and mammalian target protein signaling of rapamycin, and all of these processes are associated with epilepsy. Ong et al. found that extracellular BCAAs and glutamate were chronically elevated about 1.5–3 times higher than baseline in brain regions where seizures began and spread, and isoleucine was significantly higher than baseline as early as 3 h before the onset of spontaneous seizures, compared to regions not involved in seizures. An animal experiment has shown that the clock protein REV-ERBα regulates the chronotropic changes of GABA function by regulating the rhythmic expression of GABA transporters on neurons and glia cells, thus regulating the rhythmicity of seizures in epilepsy. Bernard et al. proposed a molecular oscillation and rhythmic hypothesis of epilepsy, the core of which is the 24-h oscillation of gene and protein expression in different cells and organs throughout the body. Molecular oscillations control the rhythm of many physiological activities, and the study of molecular oscillations may help to understand the mechanism of epilepsy and search for new predictive biomarkers.

Other scenarios: Multiple studies have confirmed that it is possible to use an electronic diary to predict seizure risk over a 24-h period based on the user's self-predictions. The likelihood of future seizures can also be predicted based on the seizure cycle determined by the seizure diary. In environmental terms, weather changes are one of the most significant environmental risk factors for seizures, as increased neuronal activity correlates with increased temperature or decreased atmospheric pressure. Rakers et al. found that low atmospheric pressure and high air humidity increased the risk of seizures, while high ambient temperature seemed to reduce the risk of seizures, although these results need to be further verified in different regions. Non-invasive seizure prediction can be achieved based on the weather combined with sleep and periodicity characteristics. In terms of hormone levels, the secretion of melatonin and cortisol has a clear circadian rhythm and is closely related to seizure development. Regarding behavior, alcohol consumption and sleep-wake cycles are also associated with the risk of seizures, and although studies have suggested that sleep efficiency decreases before seizures, the specific relationship between sleep and seizures remains unclear. In terms of dynamics, markers used to detect critical slowdowns can be combined with the incidence of seizure-like spikes, promising to create a powerful predictive tool.

5.3 Prevention and Management of Pregnancy Complications

Ziyi Chen

5.3.1 Obstetric Complications in Women with Epilepsy

WWE face more challenges in pregnancy due to increased risks to the mother and fetus. A review of previous retrospective studies on pregnancy outcomes and complications in women with epilepsy (including 38 studies involving 2,837,325 pregnant women) showed that women with epilepsy in pregnancy had an increased risk of spontaneous abortion, prenatal bleeding, hypertension, induction of labor, cesarean section, preterm delivery (earlier than 37 weeks of gestation), fetal growth restriction, and postpartum bleeding. However, there was no difference in gestational diabetes mellitus or fetal stillbirth. Compared with patients who do not take ASMs, patients who take ASMs have higher rates of labor induction, fetal growth restriction, and postpartum hemorrhage, and are also more likely to be admitted to neonatal care units. A comparison of patients who took monotherapy during pregnancy and those who took multiple medications for epilepsy found that patients who took multiple ASMs had an increased rate of cesarean section but no differences in other complications were observed.

In addition, studies have shown that women taking antiseizure medications and women with epilepsy have a significantly higher rate of spontaneous abortion than women not taking antiseizure medications or without epilepsy. Women taking antiseizure medications are significantly more likely to terminate their pregnancies than women not taking antiseizure medications. The prevalence of preeclampsia is higher in women with epilepsy than in women without epilepsy, and obesity is also more common in pregnant women with epilepsy than in women without epilepsy.

Therefore, obstetricians and epilepsy specialists should be aware of the increased risk of pregnancy complications in women with epilepsy during pregnancy compared with normal pregnant women and should develop preventive mechanisms and countermeasures accordingly.

5.3.2 Measures for the Management of Pregnancy Complications in Women with Epilepsy

Overall, while WWE may have a higher risk of pregnancy complications, studies show that more than 90% of WWE pregnant women do not have any significant complications, and most pregnant WWE go on to deliver healthy babies. In China, maternal health management has been included in the national basic public health service program, management programs, and related measures are complete and standardized, and pregnant women with epilepsy generally do not need additional monitoring.

Clinical Recommendations for Management of Pregnancy Complications
However, in view of the increased risk of complications during childbirth, women with epilepsy should be guided by a professional doctor. Regular antenatal check-ups for patients with epilepsy during pregnancy should be conducted by a team composed of neurologists, obstetricians, and midwives. Obstetric care and preparation before delivery should be made, and timely hospitalization should be provided if complications occur during pregnancy. For unplanned pregnancies in WWE, follow-up treatment options should be urgently discussed with a neurologist, and self-withdrawal or self-reduction of medication is not recommended. In order to reduce the occurrence of complications during pregnancy, in addition to prenatal consultation, the patient's

self-management is also very important. It is recommended that WWE take adequate rest during pregnancy, complete regular and standardized delivery check-ups, control excessive weight gain, minimize the various factors that induce seizures, and avoid voluntarily stopping or reducing the use of antiseizure medications during pregnancy.

5.4 Choice of Anesthesia and Mode of Delivery

Ziyi Chen and Leihao Sha

5.4.1 Choice of Birth Mode for Female Patients with Epilepsy

The choice of mode of delivery for women with epilepsy is a focus of pregnancy management in WWE. The Royal College of Obstetricians and Gynaecologists (RCOG) Guidelines for Epilepsy in Pregnancy state that most pregnancies in women with epilepsy are uncomplicated and the status of seizure control in women with epilepsy in pregnancy should be repeatedly assessed. A diagnosis of epilepsy is not an indication of a planned cesarean section or induction of labor. In summary, we consider WWE with well-controlled seizures to be free of potential obstetric risks for whom there is no indication of a need for early delivery. The small number of patients that experience a significant exacerbation of seizures during pregnancy, repeated seizures, and seizures of prolonged duration are at high risk of developing status epilepticus, in which case cesarean section may be considered. There is currently no evidence regarding the optimal timing and mode of delivery in WWE. Therefore, WWE should be informed that the vast majority of these women can deliver vaginally.

5.4.2 Prevention and Management of Epileptic Seizures During Delivery in Women with Epilepsy

The RCOG guidelines for the management of epilepsy in pregnancy state that women with epilepsy in pregnancy are at a lower risk of seizures during delivery and that painless delivery can be used appropriately during labor to reduce risk factors for seizures, such as insomnia, stress, and dehydration. WWE should continue to take ASMs at the time of delivery, or if they cannot take them orally, they should be delivered intravenously. Previous studies have shown that only approximately 2–4% of patients experience tonic-clonic seizures during labor or within 24 h after delivery, resulting in a lack of oxygen in the mother and fetus. Sleep deprivation and stopping taking ASMs are risk factors for seizures during labor, and pain, fatigue, stress, and dehydration may also be contributing factors. The doctor should ensure that the patient continues to take ASMs during labor, and consider intravenous administration to avoid vomiting. Proper fluid rehydration and analgesia can reduce the risk of seizures during labor.

If a seizure occurs during labor, reasonable treatment should be given promptly to avoid the occurrence of status epilepticus. Pregnant women should lie on their left side to keep the airway open and facilitate oxygenation. No studies have indicated the best treatment for seizures during labor. Benzodiazepines are the first choice medication for patients with epilepsy during pregnancy as emergency drug selection to stop prolonged ongoing seizures or status epilepticus: lorazepam 0.1 mg/kg (the dosage is less than 4 mg and can be readministered after 10–20 min) or diazepam 5–10 mg for patients with intravenous access. For patients without intravenous access, diazepam 10–20 mg is given rectally, and midazolam 5–10 mg can also be administered if the seizure lasts for 15 min and the dose can be repeated. If seizures are still not effectively controlled, use of phenytoin sodium or fosphenytoin may be considered. If the uterus continues to have high tone, drugs to suppress contractions may be given. After the mother is stable, continuous electronic fetal heart monitoring is required. If the fetal heart rate does not recover within 5 min or if the seizure occurs again, the pregnancy should be terminated. A neonatology team should be present to assist and avoid the occurrence of neonatal drug withdrawal syndrome (due to maternal benzodiazepines or ASMs).

5.4.3 Mode of Anesthesia for Women with Epilepsy

Painless delivery is very important for female patients with epilepsy. Epilepsy is not a contraindication to any mode of anesthesia or analgesia. Alternative methods include transcutaneous electrical nerve stimulation (TENS), gas anesthesia (Entonox), and regional anesthesia (epidural anesthesia, spinal anesthesia, and epidural combined spinal anesthesia). The use of pethidine for labor analgesia in women with epilepsy should be approached cautiously due to the presence of norpethidine, a metabolite of pethidine, and seizures can be induced when high doses of norpethidine are present in patients with normal renal function. In addition, diacetylmorphine is superior to pethidine for analgesia during labor. Etomidate should also be avoided due to seizuregenic tedencies. And sevoflurane should avoid use of a high dose (>1.5 minimum alveolar concentration) to limit pro-convulsant properties.

WWE anesthesia options during delivery:

For patients with frequent seizures and no obvious cause, general anesthesia is preferred, and specific drug options are as follows:

1. Propofol, non-depolarizing muscle relaxants such as vecuronium bromide and rocuronium bromide are the main anesthesia induction agents. Analgesia used is mainly remifentanil, benzodiazepines such as midazolam can be used after delivery of the fetus, and the dosage can be increased, and opioids used can include fentanyl or sufentanil.
2. Cis-atracurium or meperidine are relatively prohibited, and their metabolites have epileptogenic effects.

3. After the end of general anesthesia, neostigmine is prohibited, because it is easy to result in retrograde anti-cholinesterase activity, acetylcholine accumulation, and M-like as well as N-like effects, leading to muscle tremors and seizures induction.

For patients who can cooperate and have good epilepsy control, intravertebral anesthesia can be used. For patients who choose vaginal delivery, preoperative assessment and preparation for immediate cesarean section, epidural or lumbo-epidural analgesia can be selected.

5.5 Antiseizure Medications in Pregnancy

Zhenlei Wang

5.5.1 Changes in the Concentration of Different Antiseizure Medications During Pregnancy

There are different rules for changes in blood concentration of antiseizure medications during pregnancy between traditional and new ASMs. Among the traditional ASMs, the concentration of phenytoin (PHT) decreases significantly, and the highest clearance rate and the lowest concentration occurs in the third trimester, while levels of carbamazepine (CBZ), phenobarbital (PB), and valproic acid (VPA) fluctuate less. The second generation ASMs such as lamotrigine (LTG), levetiracetam (LEV), oxcarbazepine (OXC), topiramate (TPM), and zonisamide (ZNS) show more obvious fluctuations during pregnancy, and the peak clearance rate and the lowest concentration of these occurs in the second trimester. The serum concentrations of LEV, TPM, and OXC can be reduced by 30–50%, and the decrease of LTG can even be as high as 70%. As a result, patients who use new ASMs such as LEV, LTG, TPM, or OXC have a higher rate of poor seizure control during pregnancy. In the case of LTG, which is currently the most commonly used ASM during pregnancy, higher quality studies have established that a 35% decrease in concentration and a 60% decrease in the ratio of concentration to dose are associated with a significant increase in the frequency of seizures during pregnancy (see Table 5.2 for details of the fluctuations in concentration and clearance of the various drugs mentioned above during pregnancy.) (Duan et al. 2022).

5.5.2 Causes of Concentration Changes of Antiseizure Medications in Pregnancy

Pregnancy is a special period that women with epilepsy can experience. Due to particular physiological changes that occur in pregnancy, medication and blood

Table 5.2 Changes in concentration and clearance of antiseizure medications during pregnancy

Antiseizure medications	Gestational change	
	Concentration fluctuations	Fluctuations in clearance
CBZ	Total concentration decreased by 9% in the second trimester and 12% in the third trimester. There was no change in free concentration. The total concentration and free concentration of the main active product 10, 11-epoxy carbamazepine (CBZ-EPO) had no significant change	The clearance rates of total CBZ and total/free CBZ-EPO were not significantly changed. The clearance of free CBZ increased slightly
PB	Total concentration decreases by 47% in the third trimester	Increased by 25% in the third trimester
PTH	Total concentration decreased by 56–61% during pregnancy, while free concentration decreased by 16–31%	The concentration increased by 117% during pregnancy
VPA	Dose/concentration ratio (DCR) reduced by 46%	Apparent clearance increased, while intrinsic clearance did not change significantly
LTG	The CDR of LTG during pregnancy was about 34% of the non-gestational baseline, and the DCR was 2.5 times higher than the baseline	It increased significantly during gestation, with an increase of 89%, 191%, and 140% in the first, middle, and third trimesters of pregnancy, respectively. Free LTG clearance increased by 89%
LEV	The concentration decreased significantly, most significantly during the third trimester; CDR decreased by 55%, and twice the dose was needed to maintain the prepregnancy blood concentration	The peak was reached in the first trimester and remained above baseline throughout the pregnancy, averaging 269% of baseline
OXC	OXC and its active metabolite monohydroxycarbamazil (MHD) will be 30–40% in blood concentration. The CDR of MHD decreased by 26.2%, 36.5%, and 38.2% in the first, middle, and third trimesters of pregnancy, respectively, and 1.5 times the dose was needed to maintain the prepregnancy blood concentration	MHD clearance increased and peaked at 138–193% of baseline in the second trimester and remained higher than baseline in the third trimester
TPM	The concentration decreases by 30–40%, with the greatest decrease in the second and third trimester of pregnancy; CDR decreased by 30% and 34% in the middle and third trimesters, respectively, and an average dose increase of 42% and 52% was needed to maintain prepregnancy blood concentration	It peaked at 139% of baseline in the second trimester and remained above baseline in the third trimester
ZNS	Concentration decreased by 25–50%, and CDR decreased by >40%, which is similar to the decrease in other ASMs	An increase of approximately 142%

concentration changes can be affected. Pregnancy is accompanied by increased drug distribution volume, increase in renal blood flow, liver metabolism induction, hormone level changes, serum protein concentration reduction, and other special physiological states that can affect the absorption, distribution, metabolism, and clearance of anti-epileptic drugs. This results in changes in the blood concentration of ASMs during pregnancy relative to before pregnancy, with varying degrees of reduction (Duan et al. 2022).

There are many factors that affect the change of blood drug concentration in WWE during pregnancy, including:

1. Maternal factors: During pregnancy, the mother experiences complex physiological changes, such as an increase of body fat and circulating blood volume, changes in hormone levels, and changes in gastrointestinal dynamics. There are complex interactions among these factors, resulting in an increase of drug clearance and a decrease in drug concentrations during pregnancy. The increase of distribution volume or the decrease of serum albumin leads to a decrease in the total concentration of high-protein binding antiseizure medications (such as phenytoin and valproic acid); increased renal blood flow resulting in decreased serum concentrations of gabapentin, pregabalin, vigabatrin, levetiracetam, and zonisamide; liver oxidation and binding enzyme induction resulting in decreased concentrations of the active components of lamotrigine, valproic acid, zonisamide, and oxcarbazepine. Nausea or vomiting during pregnancy will also affect absorption of the drugs.
2. Placental factors: The placenta also has a certain impact on drug transport and metabolism. There are many drug metabolizing enzymes in the placenta, and the placenta can also affect maternal drug metabolism by secreting hormones that affect maternal levels. In addition, many drug transporters are present in the placenta, and their expression and function can change over the course of pregnancy. For example, the expression of ABCB1 (coding P-gp) decreases from the early gestation period, and the expression of ABCC2 (coding MRP2) increases with increasing gestation.
3. Dietary factors: The influence of diet on ASM concentration during pregnancy is caused by consumption on the one hand and food composition on the other. The effect of eating is mostly non-specific, which is caused by gastrointestinal activities, such as changes in gastric emptying dynamics, increased intestinal bile concentration, or increased liver perfusion. Current studies have shown that eating can prolong the Tmax of VPA and LEV, and a high-fat diet can increase CBZ absorption. For those taking PB, a fasting diet is significantly beneficial to its absorption. A high-protein diet can increase pancreatic secretion, increase intestinal fluid volume, theoretically dilute drug concentration, and reduce Cmax, delaying drug absorption. Carbohydrates may cause a large amount of water in the small intestine to be absorbed, which may increase the concentration of drugs in the intestine. Fat can stimulate the pancreas and bile secretion, increasing the dissolution and absorption of fat-soluble drugs.

5.5.3 Current Status and Development Trends of Antiseizure Medication Concentration Monitoring

From the current situation and development trends, the monitoring of epilepsy drug concentration includes at least four levels. The first level is therapeutic drug monitoring (TDM). Traditional TDM focuses on whether the concentration of the drug meets requirements, by exploring drug processing in the body and according to the individual treatment of the patient to adjust the dose. The second level is the population pharmacokinetics (PopPK) analysis of drug concentrations in epilepsy. PopPK mainly uses nonlinear mixed-effects modeling (NONMEM) to analyze pharmacokinetic data. While the traditional epilepsy TDM mainly focuses on whether the drug concentration meets requirements, PopPK can identify and quantify covariates that affect the population pharmacokinetic parameters while obtaining the population typical values. Population pharmacokinetic analysis can effectively integrate multiple clinical study data sources, while expressing pharmacokinetic behavior of drugs in vivo, obtaining the population typical values of pharmacokinetic parameters and their variations, and interpret and quantify the influencing factors and random effects of pharmacokinetic differences between individuals. This is currently a widely used quantitative analysis method (Kanner and Bicchi 2022).

The third level of antiseizure medication concentration monitoring is population pharmacokinetic/pharmacodynamic (PopPK/PD) analysis and dose–expose–response relationship (E-R) analysis. PopPK/PD and E-R analysis are related concepts. The pharmacokinetic/pharmacodynamic model is generally established by first building a population pharmacokinetic model and then adding pharmacodynamic data to build a pharmacokinetic/pharmacodynamic model. Population analysis with a nonlinear mixed-effect model makes it possible to derive the population mean values and the variability of pharmacokinetic and pharmacodynamic parameters simultaneously. However, after constructing a population pharmacokinetic model, it is sometimes not enough to construct a population pharmacokinetic/pharmacodynamic model, and in these cases, E-R analysis can be performed by regression. E-R analysis refers to the relationship between dose and effect after drug administration, described as the relationship between the dose, the amount of exposure observed in terms of systemic drug concentration or drug concentration at the site of action, and the pharmacodynamic effect caused by the drug exposure and the resulting efficacy or safety. In addition, PopPK/PD and E-R analysis can evaluate the effect of multiple relevant intrinsic and extrinsic factors (covariates) on drug concentrations and other clinical endpoints obtained from a large number of subjects with a wide range of backgrounds, while reducing stress on subjects by reducing the frequency of sampling (optimal sampling) of individual subjects. With the rapid globalization of drug concentration monitoring, population analysis has become a valuable analytical method to evaluate and analyze racial differences in patient pharmacokinetic characteristics as well as to evaluate appropriate dosages and dosing.

The fourth level of epilepsy drug concentration monitoring is mechanically-intelligent detection based on physiologically based pharmacokinetics (PBPK) and artificial intelligence (AI). Based on the PBPK model, the pharmacokinetic behavior of drugs is described from the mechanistic perspective by integrating physiological characteristics, population characteristics, drug active ingredients and preparation characteristics, which supports the predictive ability of pharmacokinetics. As a mechanistic model, physiology-based pharmacokinetic models can help individual medication decisions in patients with epilepsy by summarizing existing knowledge and data and combining one or more sources of evidence related to model analysis. AI is an emerging science that researches and develops theoretical methods and application systems for simulating, extending, and expanding human intelligence. AI develops and uses complex computer algorithms to perform tasks normally required of humans, such as visual perception, pattern recognition, decision-making, and problem solving. Currently, AI is widely used in medical fields such as medical imaging, pathological diagnosis, drug research and development, and health management. With the advent of the era of medical big data, clinically proven AI technology can play an increasingly important role in precision medicine. AI mainly includes pattern recognition, machine learning, data mining, and intelligent algorithms. Machine learning (ML) is an important branch of AI. ML simulates the way humans learn, relying on existing data or past experiences, using advanced algorithms to infer the computer's own logical rules, and finally making predictions and supporting decisions. There are many kinds of algorithms used in ML. The classic algorithms in the medical field include artificial neural networks, decision trees, gradient lifting decision trees, extreme trees, and support vector machines. Overall, AI is an empirical "modeling and simulation" approach that takes into account the disease course as well as drug and patient characteristics to accurately predict drug efficacy and thus determine the best individualized drug treatment plan for the patient. Different machine learning algorithms have their own advantages and disadvantages. However, it is still unclear which algorithm has the best predictive performance. In addition, the reported algorithms still lack rigorous clinical validation and widespread adoption is difficult.

No matter what level of epilepsy drug concentration monitoring is used, one encounters the need to determine drug concentration, the standard of drug concentration, and the individualized treatment of epilepsy patients from different teams. Generally speaking, the determination of drug concentration is completed in the central laboratory of a hospital, and the detection ability of the central laboratory that undertakes the determination of the concentration of epilepsy drugs and the detection ability of the standard setting team of drug concentration standards may be different. To this end, in order to ensure the testing capacity of the central laboratory and the international consistency of testing data, the International Accreditation Forum (IAF) and International Laboratory Accreditation Cooperation (ILAC) have established a mature international system for the consistency of drug concentration testing. The IAF is a joint initiative of the American National Standard Institute (ANSI) and the Registrar Accreditation Board (RAB) and is an international cooperative organization composed of conformity assessment accreditation bodies worldwide and other relevant bodies interested in engaging in conformity assessment activities in management systems, products, services, people and other similar areas. The ILAC was founded in 1978 and its purpose is to improve the acceptance of testing and calibration results issued by accredited laboratories, in order to establish international cooperation in the promotion of international trade.

The current international standard for mutual recognition of laboratory competence for testing concentrations of epilepsy drugs is ISO/IEC 17025:2018 "General Requirements for Laboratory Competence for Testing and Calibration." In China, it is equivalent to the China National Accreditation Service for Conformity Assessment (CNAS)-CL01 "Standards for Accreditation of Testing and Calibration Laboratory Competence." CNAS is a national accreditation body approved and authorized by the Certification and Accreditation Administration according to the provisions of the Certification and Accreditation Regulations of the People's Republic of China and is uniformly responsible for the accreditation of certification bodies, laboratories, inspection bodies, and other related bodies. Therefore, for the specific implementation of epilepsy drug concentration detection of the central laboratory and drug concentration standards formulated by the unit or organization if not from the same unit, it is recommended to use IAF-MLA/CNAS- or ILAC-MRA/CNAS-accredited laboratories that issue drug concentration test results.

5.5.4 Monitoring of ASM Concentration and Population Analysis of Drug Effects

PopPK, PopPK/PD, E-R analysis, and other similar technical means belong to the group of population analysis techniques for epilepsy drug concentration monitoring. PopPK can help to identify covariates that significantly influence PK variability and provide guidance for individualized drug delivery regimens for patients with epilepsy. For example, when a strong association between body weight and drug exposure is observed, dosing by body weight or grouping by body weight may be supported. In specific clinical practice, PopPK analysis should also be combined with a good understanding of the relationship between drug exposure and drug efficacy, target occupancy, or drug toxicity to co-guide or further optimize the dosing regimen. In addition, PopPK can simulate drug exposure levels under untested or off-label dosing regimens. For example, PopPK can predict changes in exposure due to changes in dosage or frequency of dosing. In rare cases where this is warranted, such analyses may be used in conjunction with PopPK/PD or E-R analysis data for dosing regimens that have not been directly evaluated in clinical trials.

A key element of population analysis is the collection of covariate information. The selection of covariate index, the breadth of information distribution, and the sample size of the included population are the important bases of group PK. Covariates of population PK research should generally include demographic information of the subject population (such as race, gender, body weight, and body surface area). At the same time, relevant covariate information should be collected according to the research purpose, such as laboratory detection indicators (including liver and renal function indicators and blood tests), concomitant drugs, genetic information (including genotype), and pathological information (including disease type, severity, history of disease, and complications). Blind screening of covariates should be avoided, and it is recommended to design and investigate based on the actual clinical situation, mechanism of drug action, physiological and clinical pharmacological considerations, and study purpose. When the distribution of a covariate in a PopPK study is narrow (for continuous covariates), the sample size of subjects in a class is insufficient (for categorical covariates), or when covariates data are underrepresented, PopPK results may not fully support the effect of the covariates on drug exposure. At present, multiple continuous covariates have defined critical values (such as age and body weight) for different grades. If dose adjustment is considered based on different grades, the scope of data collection for continuous covariates should cover all target grades, not just the upper or lower end. An increase in the range and frequency of the covariate distribution generally increases the probability of finding a clinically significant covariate and decreases the likelihood of false positives for the covariate.

The main target of PopPK research is the original drug, but when the metabolite is active, the level of metabolite is high, or it affects the exposure-response relationship of the drug, the PK characteristics of its metabolites should be studied at the same time. For drugs with high-protein binding rate, it is recommended to consider the study of PK characteristics of free drugs. Indicators of PopPK studies include, but are not limited to, exposure to drugs in systemic circulation, exposure to drugs in other biological samples (such as urine, saliva, cerebrospinal fluid, and target organs or tissues), and exposure obtained by quantifying drug concentrations in tissues through imaging methods. The precision and error of PK parameters in PopPK studies depend on a variety of factors, including the total sample size of subjects, the sample size of individual sampling sites, and sampling design. Typically, the sampling time window for samples in a population PK study can be designed based on the operability of execution (such as PK sampling in a patient population) and is generally wider than in a conventional pharmacokinetic study. However, in actual practice, it is equally necessary to accurately record the actual dosing time and blood collection time. The recording requirements of drug administration before sampling can be designed with comprehensive consideration of information such as the clearance half-life of the drug. If the effects of companion drugs need to be assessed, the dosing information of these drugs should also be collected.

The design of sampling schedules is particularly important when the sample size of individual subjects' sampling sites is limited. It is recommended to design the PK sampling schedule prospectively according to the research purpose and drug characteristics to improve the reliability and reference value of PopPK research results. The following are some sampling design strategies, one or a combination of which can be selected according to the study purpose and operational feasibility: (1) Randomly assign the sampling time based on optimal design to the subjects. The sample size and sampling time of a single subject should also be determined based on the optimal design method. (2) Each subject will randomly contribute two or more samples, and the total sample can cover the entire dosing interval when used together. (3) Most subjects will take one sample at a specified time point, usually the trough concentration before administration. (4) Intensive sampling of a representative part of the patients is conducive to the establishment of the structural model.

In practice, investigators are encouraged to collect PK data from all subjects enrolled in PopPK studies. The specific sampling design depends on the intended use of the data. For example, if C_{max} is to be used in subsequent E-R analyses, consider selecting a time window covering T_{max} to obtain sufficient samples within this range. Attention should be paid to the cause of the missing PK data and whether the missing data is random or related to disease progression and drug therapy (for example, whether it is caused by patients dropping out due to lack of efficacy or adverse events). When inter-occasion variability (IOV) is large, ignoring its effects and not calculating them may affect the accurate estimation of covariates, intra-individual variability, and interindividual variability. The design of the experiment should consider sampling enough individual subjects in more than one scene to ensure that at least a moderately sized subset of subjects can provide data for each scene to estimate the inter-scene variation.

Another frequent problem in monitoring epileptic drug concentrations is missing values. Missing values may be due to the absence of data on certain drug concentrations or covariates, or may be caused by a lack of clinical effects, and needs to be analyzed in conjunction with specific cases. It is suggested to focus on whether the occurrence of missing values is random and special attention should be paid (Kiral-Kornek et al. 2018) to when the occurrence frequency of missing values increases significantly in specific populations or special scenarios. Improper handling of missing values may lead to estimation bias, which may lead to incorrect conclusions. In clinical practice, it is recommended that appropriate measures be taken to minimize missing values. In addition, missing values may complicate the interpretation of the analysis results, and the treatment of missing values should be considered in advance in the analysis plan, and studies such as sensitivity analysis should be carried out as necessary to examine the impact of missing values. In addition to missing values, data below the lower limit of quantitation and outliers may also be encountered in therapeutic drug monitoring.

Directly removing concentration values below the lower limit of quantitation (LLOQ) from analytical data may lead to bias in parameter estimates. It is recommended to select an appropriate method to deal with concentrations below LLOQ according to the characteristics of the analyzed data and the purpose of the study. The definition and reason of outliers should be clearly stated in the analysis plan. The investigator should pay attention to and distinguish between outliers. In the model development process, it is sometimes possible to consider eliminating individual data points suspected of being outliers, but it is recommended to conduct a sensitivity analysis of outliers using the final model, based on the comparison of model results with/without outliers, to examine the impact of outliers on the final parameter estimation and to describe it in the final analysis report. Excluding outliers is generally not recommended, except for outliers due to protocol violations or other human errors. For PopPK studies conducted after the exclusion of outliers, it is recommended to explain the reason for data exclusion from the perspective of physiological and clinical trial-related events.

Since PopPK's underlying model is able to obtain important features of the drug time curve, this is sufficient to make basic inferences about exposure levels and variability (interindividual, interweekly, and residual). Once the PopPK base model has been defined, further covariate modeling (in addition to structural covariates already included in the base model) can be undertaken to examine factors that further explain the origin of interindividual variation (IIV), such as demography, pathophysiology, environment, or co-medication. At all stages of model development (the base model stage, the full covariate model stage, and the final model stage), the model should be evaluated using the following criteria: (1) Successful convergence. The analyst must develop a model capable of achieving successful convergence. (2) Diagnostic graphs for visual tests. In general, tests can be classified according to the type of variable plotted or measured, as follows: Tests based on predictions (agreement graphs), for example, predicted values for the population (PRED), and predicted values for the individual (IPRED); those based on residual tests, including weighted residuals (WRES), conditional weighted residuals (CWRES), and individual weighted residuals (IWRES); tests based on parameters or empirical EBE (Bayesian estimates); and tests based on simulations. (3) LRT (Likelihood ratio test). Although the LRT is a method for evaluating nested models, it is not recommended to use LRT as the sole criterion for selection of the structure-based model due to its ability to increase type I errors. The question of how much the value of the objective function (OFV) changes as parameters are added to the model is often debated. Maximum likelihood theory states that the OFV difference of nested models is χ^2 distributed, with degrees of freedom (df) equal to the difference in the number of parameters between the models. It has been shown that such assumptions can be predictive as methodologically dependent (at least in NONMEM), and generally do not retain a nominal type I error rate. For this reason, analysts should avoid using statistical significance tests including the use of p-values, for example, to describe the differences between nested models. Although the LRT is not recommended for judging model differences, this does not mean that the size of the OFV difference is unimportant. As a general rule, an OFV change greater than 10 when an additional parameter is added is often likely to be associated with an improvement in model fit. This criterion can be relaxed to a smaller value if there is a strong biological/physiological mechanism involved that requires a particular parameter to be added to the model. For non-nested models, analysts can use methods similar to OFV values, such as Akaike information content criteria (AIC), to assess the differences between different models. The AIC value is plotted by the formula OFV + 2 * p, where p is the number of estimated parameters in the model. A model with a lower AIC value is considered superior.

In general, PopPK is the basis of population analysis, and PopPK/PD and E-R analysis are of greater clinical significance. For example, PopPK analysis generates corresponding exposure indicators, such as area under the curve (AUC_{ss}), average concentration (C_{avg_ss}), peak concentration (C_{max_ss}) or valley concentration (C_{trough_ss}) in the steady state. These exposure indicators can be comprehensively analyzed with the efficacy indicators. The efficacy indicators should be selected with full consideration of the analysis purpose and different stages of the study, including but not limited to biomarkers, surrogate endpoints, and clinical endpoints (clinical benefit endpoints or clinical outcome endpoints). Biomarker indicators are considered to be measures of physiology, pathology, or anatomy in normal physiological or pathophysiological processes, including measures suggesting disease etiology, disease susceptibility or process, measures related to therapeutic effect mechanisms, and actual clinical effects of therapeutic interventions. Different biomarkers are not closely related to the expected therapeutic effect or clinical outcome, and in general, biomarkers are not considered as endpoints for determining the efficacy and safety of new drugs. Surrogate endpoints are generally laboratory measurements or indicators of signs used in therapeutic clinical trials that have been well validated as surrogates for clinically meaningful endpoints that predict efficacy or safety/toxicity, with consistent results across multiple contexts. Clinical endpoints are variables that reflect patient sensation, function, or survival. They are the expected effect of a therapeutic intervention and are the most reliable measures of effect in clinical trials.

Quantitative data used in clinical studies, such as measured values, binary data (valid or invalid), and qualitative data such as ordered classification data, can also be used as efficacy indicators. For response measures, observations or endpoints that characterize efficacy or safety should be selected according to the purpose of the analysis. For evaluating the efficacy or safety of a drug, it is useful to analyze using clinical or surrogate endpoints as response measures. In addition, the presence or absence of adverse events is occasionally used as binary data as an indicator of a safety response. The occurrence of adverse events can provide more useful information if the analysis is disaggregated based on severity, severity, whether it is an adverse event requiring special attention, or if the analysis is performed using quantitative data such as clinical laboratory test data, depending on the purpose of the analysis. In principle, missing data on efficacy measures should be treated in the same way as the efficacy analysis and safety analysis for each clinical study. It is important to note that an accurate understanding of the characteristics of the data is the starting point for an adequate analysis before performing an exposure-effect analysis. For evaluation of the expose-effect relationship, an exploratory graphical analysis is performed prior to analysis and an overview of the observed data is obtained. This informs the assumptions considered in the analysis. It is important to calculate the aggregate measures of various factors such as covariate candidates and, by graphing the data, to understand the shape and characteristics of the distribution. Depending on the purpose of the analysis, it may be sufficient to evaluate the expose-effect relationship by graphical analysis alone.

5.5.5 ASMs Concentration Monitoring and Model-Based Precision Medicine

In May 2016, the concept of model-informed precision dosing (MIPD) was formally proposed at a medical summit in Manchester, UK. Precision medicine is a complex and difficult task, which requires multidisciplinary knowledge of diagnostics, clinical pharmacology, pharmacotherapeutics, pharmacogenomics, immunology, and cell biology to develop a drug delivery regimen tailored to the individual patient based on clinical evidence. MIPD can quantitatively analyze the impact of individual differences on drug PK/PD, and formulate the best individualized drug delivery regimen based on the individual characteristics and treatment goals of the patient. MIPD is an important part of precision medicine. One of the ultimate goals of MIPD is to use modeling and simulation technology to make accurate clinical medication regimen for patients, and this key step is inseparable from the development and application of clinical decision support systems (CDSS).

At present, PK/PD is the most used and most mature method, and the majority of the existing CDSSs are based on the principle of group PK/PD. Related professional software such as NONMEM, Phoenix NLME, Lixoft, and MATLAB, although associated with powerful modeling and computing functions to realize the prediction of individualized drug treatment plans, are difficult to use, and need a long time for user learning and training, and thus for most clinicians it is not easy to popularize and promote these software. In recent years, domestic and foreign scholars and research institutions have developed a number of CDSSs, mainly including computer platforms, web platforms, and mobile device applications (APPs) in three forms. On the whole, CDSS computer platforms have the best universal properties, followed by network platforms, with mobile device applications lagging behind. Due to the limitations of the operating platform, the functions of data management and report generation of mobile device applications are the weakest. In terms of professional attributes, the scores of web platform and computer platform are essentially equal, while mobile device applications are weaker than the first two, mainly in the aspects of drug models, dosing protocol formulation, and mapping, where there are significant gaps.

At present, MIPD and its auxiliary decision-making system has not been widely used in daily clinical practice, mainly for the following reasons: (1) the evidence base of prospective, multi-center, large-sample randomized controlled trials is insufficient, which limits the recognition and acceptance of CDSSs by general professionals and also affects the health economics evaluation of CDSS; (2) the process of incorporating CDSSs into clinical work is complicated, and the implementation process involves follow-up evaluation, sample collection and testing, drug administration plan formulation, information exchange, patient privacy protection, patient informed consent, off-label drug use, and other aspects. It requires the close cooperation of doctors, pharmacists, nursing, laboratory testing, hospital management, and other multidisciplinary teams to formulate relevant standard procedures and institutional norms; (3) The scientific and reliable certification and supervision of CDSSs requires communication and cooperation among CDSS suppliers, purchasers (such as hospital managers), users (such as clinicians, clinical pharmacists, and clinical pharmacologists), service objects (patients), and government regulatory agencies to formulate targeted technical guidelines and norms to build a favorable environment for CDSS development and application. However, there is reason to believe that with the innovation of sample collection and analysis technology, such as bedside detection, wearables, home sampling devices, biosensors, paper spray mass spectrometry and nanotechnology, as well as the development and popularization of advanced modeling and analysis methods, increasingly easy-to-use, computationally accurate, and reliable CDSS covering multiple drugs will be available, and more patients will therefore benefit from this technology.

5.5.6 Therapeutic Drug Monitoring of Antiseizure Medications

In recent years, the techniques widely used in the therapeutic drug monitoring of ASMs include high performance liquid chromatography (HPLC), high performance liquid chromatography-mass spectrometry (HPLC-MS), fluorescence polarization immunoassay (FPIA), enzyme-linked immunoassay (ELISA), and radioimmunoassay (RIA). HPLC-MS is currently a commonly used concentration detection method for ASMs. Liquid chromatography with high separation ability for complex samples is used as the separation system, and mass spectrometry with high selectivity and high sensitivity is used as the detection system. Combined with the advantages of liquid chromatography and mass spectrometry, it can provide relative molecular mass and structure information at the same time, so that its application in TDM is gradually increasing. Its specific advantages are: (1) high specificity and sensitivity; (2) can simultaneously determine dozens of substances to be measured; (3) suitable for different biological substrates; (4) wide quantitative dynamic range; (5) low average cost per time; (6) strong scalability. Compared with FPIA, which requires a special kit purchase, HPLC-MS has a relatively low operating cost despite the high price of the instrument equipment, and has the advantage of simultaneously detecting multiple substances, high specificity, and is not affected by metabolites or other drugs.

At present, the biological substrates that can be used to monitor the concentration of ASMs include: serum/plasma concentration, serum free concentration, saliva drug concentration, hair drug concentration, urine drug concentration, milk drug concentration, tear drug concentration, etc. Serum/plasma therapeutic drug monitoring is the most commonly used in clinic. With the increasing attention to free drug concentration, salivary therapeutic drug monitoring reflecting free drug concentration has become a new research field. The selection of specific detection methods should be determined according to the specific conditions of patients, with the purpose of achieving safe, scientific, reliable and convenient detection, and providing guidance and theoretical basis for the formulation of individualized treatment methods, the expansion of efficacy, the reduction of adverse reactions, and the adjustment of drug dosage.

Detection of serum/plasma concentration by HPLC or ELISA kit is the most commonly used therapeutic drug monitoring method for ASMs. Both these methods should be conducted in the center labs of hospitals by the professional operators, which needs the hospital registration and long time to wait for the final detection report. This issues directly cause the extreme poor experience feeling of the patients and hinder the wide application of therapeutic drug monitoring. Intrinsically, these actual detection conditions determine the traditional methods cannot be performed out of the hospitals and hinder the accurate, effective, and timely adjustment the medications based on the physical fitness of the patients. In this case, the development of a simple method for rapid and easy judgment of ASM concentration is of great clinical significance for the therapy. Colloidal gold labeled flow strip (LFS) have been widely utilized in rapid clinical diagnosis especially for the most well-known home-test of early pregnancy and various other fields. In this context, some studies have established LFS detection methods for ASMs, mainly LTG. At present, researchers have designed a LFS with multi test lines of different detection limits for the rapid and direct interpretation of LTG concentration range in serum. Our team has previously found that the concentration of ASMs in saliva and blood is linearly correlated. And combined with colloidal gold technology, our team further constructed a semi-quantitative detection method of LTG saliva concentration based on saliva to achieve real-time detection of LTG concentration at home.

5.6 Maternal and Fetal Risks with Seizures During Pregnancy

Leihao Sha

Seizures during pregnancy can pose significant risks to both the mother and the fetus. Convulsions are dangerous for women with epilepsy not only because they increase the risk of seizure-related falls and severe trauma, but also because they can harm the fetus due to hypoxemia and hypoxia. Focal seizures that do not progress to convulsions are assumed to have minimal influence on the fetus. However, anecdotal data suggests that they can cause transitory fetal distress, with heart rate slowing lasting up to 2.5 min. When a pregnant woman experiences seizures, it can lead to various complications and risks. One of the primary concerns is the potential harm to the fetus. Seizures can disrupt the oxygen supply to the baby, leading to fetal distress and even intrauterine growth restriction. In severe cases, seizures can result in preterm birth or stillbirth, posing a grave threat to the life of the unborn child.

Furthermore, maternal seizures can also have detrimental effects on the mother's health. Seizures during pregnancy may increase the risk of maternal injuries, such as falls or accidents during a seizure episode. Additionally, uncontrolled seizures can elevate the mother's blood pressure, putting her at risk of developing conditions like preeclampsia or eclampsia, which can be life-threatening if not managed promptly.

Managing seizures during pregnancy requires a multidisciplinary approach involving close monitoring by healthcare providers. It is essential for pregnant women with epilepsy or a history of seizures to work closely with their healthcare team to develop a comprehensive management plan that ensures the safety of both the mother and the fetus. During labor and delivery, the frequency of seizures may rise, but this is observed in only 1–2% of pregnancies in women with epilepsy. The majority of women with epilepsy will not see a change in seizure frequency during pregnancy.

5.7 Perinatal Counseling for Women with Epilepsy

Ziyi Chen

Since women with epilepsy face special fertility risks, WWE need to carry out pre-pregnancy assessment and select the best time to conceive before pregnancy to reduce the risk of fetal abnormalities and intellectual development disorders in their offspring. It is recommended that women of childbearing age with the intention to become pregnant consult with epilepsy specialists and obstetricians, so that the doctors can explain the impact of seizures themselves and ASMs on female fertility, and inform WWE of the obstetric complications related to seizures. In addition, patients with a family history of epilepsy need to be evaluated for hereditary epilepsy, and if a high genetic risk is identified, it is recommended to consult a geneticist for genetic counseling before making pregnancy decisions.

For pregnant WWE, regardless of whether the pregnancy is planned or not, if the patient is not able to reduce or withdraw their ASMs before pregnancy, she should continue to take medication regularly during pregnancy and go to the epilepsy department and obstetric clinic following conception and attend regular follow-up visits. The patient should take the initiative to record their own seizure and medication status, follow the doctor's advice to take medication regularly, and should not stop or reduce medications without authorization. Otherwise, it may lead to epilepsy recurrence or exacerbation. In addition, given the short golden age for women to have children and the low risk of teratogenicity for most low-dose ASMs, it is not clinically recommended to stop taking the drug completely before becoming pregnant, but to make adjustments depending on the patient's specific situation, for example: changing to a low-dose monotherapy, replacing a drug with a high teratogenic rate, or maintaining the original regimen but reducing the dose. At the same time, in order to ensure the stability of ASM concentration during pregnancy, blood drug concentration should be regularly monitored during pregnancy.

With regard to the choice of delivery method, patients should be informed that the vast majority of them can have a vaginal birth, and only a small number of patients with poor epileptic control or patients with a higher risk of status epilepticus need to have a cesarean section under the evaluation of a specialist.

Pain relief during delivery is of paramount importance to WWE because painful stimuli during delivery can trigger seizures that can harm the mother and fetus. However, sedation and anesthesia carry risks for both mother and fetus. Respiratory depression and aspiration pneumonia are major risk factors for maternal death. Therefore, the choice of anesthetic drugs for labor analgesia in WWE should be carefully considered.

Clinical Recommendations for Perinatal Counseling

For patients who use antiseizure medications for a long time, the selection of anesthetics in these individuals should be careful. Most antiseizure medications are liver metabolic enzyme promoters, and long-term use of liver drug enzyme activity increases, drug metabolism in the liver increases, so that the effective concentration of drugs in their original form is weakened, the duration of effect is shortened, and the effective effect concentration of their metabolites is enhanced, the duration can be prolonged, and potential side effects can increase. In addition, most antiseizure medications are central depressants, which have synergistic effects with narcotic analgesics and sedatives. When considering the use of some inhaled anesthetics (such as methoxyflurane), it is necessary to know whether the patient has liver insufficiency and its severity. When there is severe liver insufficiency, inhaled anesthetics should be used with caution to avoid acute liver injury.

For pregnant women, there should also be concerns about the effects of anesthetics on the offspring. When anesthesia is used for sedation and pain, the fetus faces risks including hypoxia, premature delivery, and congenital malformations. Most local anesthetics are considered relatively safe during pregnancy, and since a single dose of conventional anesthetics has only minimal teratogenicity, the risk of teratogenicity should not be overstated. In addition, the risk of preterm birth is reduced because the fetal organs are already well developed and the placenta is stable during normal delivery.

References

Cook MJ, O'brien TJ, Berkovic SF, et al. Prediction of seizure likelihood with a long-term, implanted seizure advisory system in patients with drug-resistant epilepsy: a first-in-man study. Lancet Neurol. 2013;12(6):563–71. https://doi.org/10.1016/s1474-4422(13)70075-9.

Duan Y, Li W, Lai W, et al. Pharmacokinetic changes and countermeasures of antiepileptic drugs in pregnant women with epilepsy. Chin J Mod Appl Pharm. 2022;39(15):2039–44. (in Chinese).

Gabeff V, Teijeiro T, Zapater M, et al. Interpreting deep learning models for epileptic seizure detection on EEG signals. Artif Intell Med. 2021;117:102084. https://doi.org/10.1016/j.artmed.2021.102084.

Harden CL, Hopp J, Ting TY, et al. Management issues for women with epilepsy-focus on pregnancy (an evidence-based review): I. Obstetrical complications and change in seizure frequency: report of the Quality Standards Subcommittee and Therapeutics and Technology Assessment Subcommittee of the American Academy of Neurology and the American Epilepsy Society. Epilepsia. 2009;50(5):1229–36.

Kanner AM, Bicchi MM. Antiseizure medications for adults with epilepsy: a review. JAMA. 2022;327(13):1269–81. https://doi.org/10.1001/jama.2022.3880.

Kiral-Kornek I, Roy S, Nurse E, et al. Epileptic seizure prediction using big data and deep learning: toward a mobile system. EBioMedicine. 2018;27:103–11. https://doi.org/10.1016/j.ebiom.2017.11.032.

Lyu Q, Gong S, Yin J, et al. Soft wearable healthcare materials and devices. Adv Healthc Mater. 2021;10(17):e2100577. https://doi.org/10.1002/adhm.202100577.

Mckee JL, Kaufman MC, Gonzalez AK, et al. Leveraging electronic medical record-embedded standardised electroencephalogram reporting to develop neonatal seizure prediction models: a retrospective cohort study. Lancet Digit Health. 2023;5(4):e217–26. https://doi.org/10.1016/s2589-7500(23)00004-3.

Reuben C, Karoly P, Freestone DR, et al. Ensembling crowdsourced seizure prediction algorithms using long-term human intracranial EEG. Epilepsia. 2020;61(2):e7–12. https://doi.org/10.1111/epi.16418.

Sahu R, Dash SR, Cacha LA, et al. Epileptic seizure detection: a comparative study between deep and traditional machine learning techniques. J Integr Neurosci. 2020;19(1):1–9. https://doi.org/10.31083/j.jin.2020.01.24.

Suggested Readings

Abbasi B, Goldenholz DM. Machine learning applications in epilepsy. Epilepsia. 2019;60(10):2037–47. https://doi.org/10.1111/epi.16333.

Baud MO, Kleen JK, Mirro EA, et al. Multi-day rhythms modulate seizure risk in epilepsy. Nat Commun. 2018;9(1):88. https://doi.org/10.1038/s41467-017-02577-y.

Bergstrand M, Karlsson MO. Handling data below the limit of quantification in mixed effect models. AAPS J. 2009;11(2):371–80.

Byon W, Fletcher CV, Brundage RC. Impact of censoring data below an arbitrary quantification limit on structural model misspecification. J Pharmacokinet Pharmacodyn. 2008;35(1):101–16.

Darwich AS, Polasek TM, Aronson JK, et al. Model-informed precision dosing: background, requirements, validation, implementation, and forward trajectory of individualizing drug therapy. Annu Rev Pharmacol Toxicol. 2021;61:225–45.

Drug Evaluation Center, State Drug Administration. Technical guidelines for population pharmacokinetic studies. 2020. www.cde.org.cn/main/news/viewInfoCommon/b3e8205a4749caa026414514cdf45ac.

Eggleston KS, Olin BD, Fisher RS. Ictal tachycardia: the head-heart connection. Seizure. 2014;23(7):496–505. https://doi.org/10.1016/j.seizure.2014.02.012.

Epilepsy in pregnancy, in RCOG Green-top guideline no. 68. 2016.

Gao Y, Liu A, Wang L, et al. A self-interpretable deep learning model for seizure prediction using a multi-scale prototypical part network. IEEE Trans Neural Syst Rehabil Eng. 2023;31:1847–56. https://doi.org/10.1109/tnsre.2023.3260845.

Harden CL, Meador KJ, Pennell PB, et al. Management issues for women with epilepsy-focus on pregnancy (an evidence-based review): II. Teratogenesis and perinatal outcomes: report of the Quality Standards Subcommittee and Therapeutics and Technology Subcommittee of the American Academy of Neurology and the American Epilepsy Society. Epilepsia. 2009b;50(5):1237–46.

Herzog AG, Mandle HB, Maceachern DB. Association of unintended pregnancy with spontaneous fetal loss in women with epilepsy: findings of the Epilepsy Birth Control Registry. JAMA Neurol. 2019;76(1):50–5.

Hiemke C, Bergemann N, Clement HW, et al. Consensus guidelines for therapeutic drug monitoring in neuropsychopharmacology: update 2017. Pharmacopsychiatry. 2018;51(1/2):9–62.

Hogg MC, Raoof R, El Naggar H, et al. Elevation in plasma tRNA fragments precede seizures in human epilepsy. J Clin Invest. 2019;129(7):2946–51. https://doi.org/10.1172/JCI126346.

Howard J. Artificial intelligence: implications for the future of work. Am J Ind Med. 2019;62(11):917–26.

Ihle M, Feldwisch-Drentrup H, Teixeira CA, et al. EPILEPSIAE—a European epilepsy database. Comput Methods Prog Biomed. 2012;106(3):127–38. https://doi.org/10.1016/j.cmpb.2010.08.011.

Johansson ÅM, Karlsson MO. Comparison of methods for handling missing covariate data. AAPS J. 2013;15(4):1232–41.

Karasmanoglou A, Antonakakis M, Zervakis M. ECG-based semi-supervised anomaly detection for early detection and monitoring of epileptic seizures. Int J Environ Res Public Health. 2023;20(6):5000. https://doi.org/10.3390/ijerph20065000.

Keizer RJ, Jansen RS, Rosing H, et al. Incorporation of concentration data below the limit of quantification in population pharmacokinetic analyses. Pharmacol Res Perspect. 2015;3(2):e00131.

Kini LG, Davis KA, Wagenaar JB. Data integration: combined imaging and electrophysiology data in the cloud. Neuroimage. 2016;124(Pt B):1175–81. https://doi.org/10.1016/j.neuroimage.2015.05.075.

Li J, Sheng D, Chen J, et al. Artificial intelligence in breast imaging: potentials and challenges. Phys Med Biol. 2023a;68:23TR01.

Li QY, Tang BH, Wu YE, et al. Machine learning: a new approach for dose individualization. Clin Pharmacol Ther. 2023b;115:727.

Liang Z, Wu S, Yang C, et al. Portable intelligent seizure monitoring system based on Android system. J Biomed Eng. 2016;33(01):31–7.
Liu B, Zhang Y, Zhang H, et al. Selection of sedative agents in pregnant and lactating patients. Anesth Saf Qual Control. 2019;3(03):168–71. (in Chinese).
Macea J, Bhagubai M, Broux V, De Vos M, Van Paesschen W. In-hospital and home-based long-term monitoring of focal epilepsy with a wearable electroencephalographic device: diagnostic yield and user experience. Epilepsia. 2023;64(4):937–50.
Naganur V, Sivathamboo S, Chen Z, Kusmakar S, Antonic-Baker A, O'Brien TJ, Kwan P. Automated seizure detection with noninvasive wearable devices: a systematic review and meta-analysis. Epilepsia. 2022;63(8):1930–41. https://doi.org/10.1111/epi.17297.
Nickel R, Silvado CE, Germiniani FM, et al. Quality of life issues and occupational performance of persons with epilepsy. Arq Neuropsiquiatr. 2012;70(2):140–4. https://doi.org/10.1590/s0004-282x2012000200013.
Nukala U, Rodriguez Messan M, Yogurtcu ON, Wang X, Yang H. A systematic review of the efforts and hindrances of modeling and simulation of CAR T-cell therapy. AAPS J. 2021;23(3):52.
Ogungbenro K, Aarons L. Optimisation of sampling windows design for population pharmacokinetic experiments. J Pharmacokinet Pharmacodyn. 2008;35(4):465–82.
Ong C, Damisah EC, Gruenbaum SE, et al. Increased branched-chain amino acids at baseline and hours before a spontaneous seizure in the human epileptic brain. Epilepsia. 2021;62(6):e88–97. https://doi.org/10.1111/epi.16920.
Patel T, Grindrod K. Antiseizure drugs for women with epilepsy: before, during, and after pregnancy. Can Fam Physician. 2020;66(4):266–9.
Patsalos PN, Spencer EP, Berry DJ. Therapeutic drug monitoring of antiepileptic drugs in epilepsy: a 2018 update. Ther Drug Monit. 2018;40(5):526–48.
Polasek TM, Kirkpatrick C, Rostami-Hodjegan A. Precision dosing to avoid adverse drug reactions. Ther Adv Drug Saf. 2019;10:2042098619894147.
Poweleit EA, Vinks AA, Mizuno T. Artificial intelligence and machine learning approaches to facilitate therapeutic drug management and model-informed precision dosing. Ther Drug Monit. 2023;45(2):143–50.
Proix T, Truccolo W, Leguia MG, et al. Forecasting seizure risk in adults with focal epilepsy: a development and validation study. Lancet Neurol. 2021;20(2):127–35. https://doi.org/10.1016/s1474-4422(20)30396-3.
Rosas-Romero R, Guevara E, Peng K, et al. Prediction of epileptic seizures with convolutional neural networks and functional near-infrared spectroscopy signals. Comput Biol Med. 2019;111:103355. https://doi.org/10.1016/j.compbiomed.2019.103355.
Royal College of Obstetricians & Gynaecologists (RCOG). Epilepsy in pregnancy (Green-top guideline no. 68). London: Royal College of Obstetricians & Gynaecologists; 2016. https://www.rcog.org.uk/en/guidelines-researchservices/guidelines/gtg68/. Accessed 27 Apr 2021.
SIGN. Diagnosis and management of epilepsy in adults. Edinburgh: SIGN; 2015. https://www.sign.ac.uk/our-guidelines/diagnosis-and-management-ofepilepsy-in-adults/. Accessed 27 Apr 2021.
Stankevičiūtė K, Woillard JB, Peck RW, Marquet P, van der Schaar M. Bridging the worlds of pharmacometrics and machine learning. Clin Pharmacokinet. 2023;62:1551.
Stephen LJ, Harden C, Tomson T, et al. Management of epilepsy in women. Lancet Neurol. 2019;18(5):481–91.
Tomson T, Battino D, Bromley R, et al. Executive summary: management of epilepsy in pregnancy: a report from the international league against epilepsy task force on women and pregnancy. Epilepsia. 2019;60(12):2343–5.
Vinks AA, Peck RW, Neely M, Mould DR. Development and implementation of electronic health record-integrated model-informed clinical decision support tools for the precision dosing of drugs. Clin Pharmacol Ther. 2020;107(1):129–35.
Voinescu PE, Park S, Chen LQ, et al. Antiepileptic drug clearances during pregnancy and clinical implications for women with epilepsy. Neurology. 2018;91(13):e1228–36.

Weisdorf S, Duun-Henriksen J, Kjeldsen MJ, et al. Ultra-long-term subcutaneous home monitoring of epilepsy-490 days of EEG from nine patients. Epilepsia. 2019;60(11):2204–14. https://doi.org/10.1111/epi.16360.

Welfare JLa. Guideline for exposure-response analysis of drugs. 2020a. www.pref.fukuoka.lg.jp/uploaded/attachment/114730.pdf.

Welfare JLa. Guideline on population pharmacokinetic and pharmacodynamic analysis. 2020b. https://www.pmda.go.jp/files/000235608.pdf.

Xing KP. Development of wearable comprehensive tonic-clonic epilepsy monitoring system. Soochow University; 2020. (in Chinese).

Yin X, Liu Y, Guo Y, et al. Pharmacokinetic changes for newer antiepileptic drugs and seizure control during pregnancy. CNS Neurosci Ther. 2022;28(5):658–66.

Yu X. Data processing algorithm and software development based on epilepsy monitoring bracelet. Harbin Institute of Technology; 2021.

Zhang YZ. Algorithm research and circuit design of wearable seizure detection chip based on EEG. Beijing Jiaotong University; 2021.

Zhang Y, Yang S, Liu Y, et al. Integration of 24 feature types to accurately detect and predict seizures using scalp EEG signals. Sensors (Basel). 2018;18(5):1372. https://doi.org/10.3390/s18051372.

Zhang M, Qin Q, Zhang S, et al. Aerobic glycolysis imaging of epileptic foci during the inter-ictal period. EBioMedicine. 2022;79:104004. https://doi.org/10.1016/j.ebiom.2022.104004.

Folic Acid Supplementation During Pregnancy

6

Ziyi Chen, Yifei Duan, and Lei Chen

6.1 Recommendations for Folic Acid Supplementation in Current National Guidelines

Ziyi Chen

The maternal requirement for folic acid is increased during pregnancy, and the American Association of Neurology (AAN) guidelines recommend that all women with epilepsy take folic acid supplementation during pregnancy to reduce the risk of major congenital malformations. Most public health agencies currently recommend that women take a folic acid supplement of 0.4 mg/day during pregnancy to prevent neural tube defects (NTDs). However, studies have shown that ASM use may cause a further deficiency of folic acid, and that folic acid supplementation in patients who take ASMs may normalize serum folic acid concentrations, making it more desirable to take folic acid in WWE than in women who do not take ASMs.

In 2009, the ANN suggested that folic acid supplementation during pregnancy may reduce the risk of fetal abnormalities. However, there is currently no uniform conclusion on the dosage of folic acid supplementation recommended in WWE, which varies from guideline to guideline (Table 6.1).

In 1992, the U.S. Public Health Service (PHS) recommended that all women of childbearing age should take 0.4 mg of folic acid daily to prevent NTDs. The current ANN guidelines recommend folic acid supplementation: high-risk pregnant women (such as those with a family history of NTDs, previous birth of NTDs

Z. Chen
Department of Neurology, The First Affiliated Hospital, Sun Yat-sen University, Guangzhou, China
e-mail: chenziyi@mail.sysu.edu.cn

Y. Duan · L. Chen (✉)
Department of Neurology, West China Hospital, Sichuan University, Chengdu, China

L. Chen (ed.), *Women with Epilepsy in Child-bearing Age*,
https://doi.org/10.1007/978-981-97-3921-9_6

Table 6.1 Guideline recommendation for folic acid supplement for women with epilepsy

Guideline	Recommended dose	Recommended duration
SIGN 2015	Not taking any ASMs: 0.4 mg/day Taking ASMs: 5 mg/day	Before pregnancy and continues throughout the first trimester
RCOG 2016	Taking ASMs: 5 mg/day	Before pregnancy and continues throughout the first trimester
ANN/AES 2009	Taking ASMs: >0.4 mg/day	Before pregnancy and continues throughout the pregnancy
ETDP-EFA 2007	Many epilepsy experts recommend that women with epilepsy should take a higher dose of folic acid (0.8–4 mg/day)	Before pregnancy and continues throughout the pregnancy
China 2021	Not taking any ASMs: 0.4 mg/day Taking ASMs: 5 mg/day	Before pregnancy and continues throughout the pregnancy
NICE 2012 (update 2016)	5 mg/day	Before pregnancy and continues throughout the pregnancy

fetuses, and those taking ASMs), it is recommended to supplement folic acid at a dose of at least 0.4 mg/day. Since 2007, the guidelines of the Chinese Medical Association also recommend that all women of childbearing age with epilepsy should take 5 mg of folic acid per day before 3 months of pregnancy. In addition, other guidelines also include women with epilepsy in the high-risk group, recommending 5 mg/day of folic acid during pregnancy. The 2011 UK guidelines recommend that folic acid should be taken during at least the first 3 months of pregnancy, with a recommended dose of 0.4–5 mg/day. A 2013 study on the effects of ASMs on offspring neurodevelopment (NEAD) found that patients who took folic acid during pregnancy had offspring with a higher average IQ than those who were not exposed to folic acid during pregnancy. However, the study did not specify when folic acid was started, for how long, or at what dose. The 2016 RCOG guidance states that pre-pregnancy folic acid supplementation (recommended dose of 5 mg/day) may be beneficial for reducing the risk of ASM-induced cognitive impairment. The 2021 China Guidelines for the Management of Women with Epilepsy during Pregnancy recommend that women with epilepsy should take folic acid supplements daily from the time of pregnancy and continue until at least 12 weeks of pregnancy (Grade A recommendation). If the patient has not taken ASMs, the recommended daily dose of folic acid is 0.4 mg; if she takes folic acid antagonists or has a history of miscarriage, or has produced a neural tube teratoma, the recommended daily dose of folic acid is 5 mg (Grade D recommended).

6.2 Benefits and Potential Harms of Folic Acid Supplementation During Pregnancy in Women with Epilepsy

Yifei Duan

6.2.1 Benefits of Folic Acid Supplementation During Pregnancy in Women with Epilepsy

Folic acid supplementation is known to prevent fetal developmental abnormalities. In recent years, studies have found that folic acid can also prevent premature birth, miscarriage, and other adverse pregnancy outcomes.

A study of 388 pregnancy outcomes among 244 patients with epilepsy found that women who took folic acid during pregnancy had a much lower rate of spontaneous miscarriage. Among women taking folic acid supplements, spontaneous miscarriages occurred in 9 out of 160 pregnancies (5.7%), compared with 30 out of 228 pregnancies (13.2%) among women who did not take folic acid supplements. The odds ratio of spontaneous miscarriage among women who did not take folic acid was 2.6 (95% CI: 1.2–5.6, $P = 0.01$). Regarding folic acid supplementation, the low-dose pregnancy group (0.4 mg/day; $N = 33$) did not experience spontaneous abortion. All spontaneous abortions occurred in the high folic acid supplement dose group (5 mg/day; $N = 127$). Several studies have reported that folic acid supplements could be associated with better neurodevelopment in children exposed to ASMs. Children with mothers of folic acid supplements are associated with reduced risks of autism and intellectual disability compared with those without folic acid supplements. And a potential dose-dependent effect was observed in certain studies with exploratory analysis. As for congenital abnormalities, no significant associations have been observed between folic acid supplements and major congenital malformations. However, there may be a potential trend that child with mothers of folic acid supplements could be at lower risks of major congenital malformations than those without folic acid supplements (Adab et al. 2004; Meador et al. 2020; Hernandez Diaz et al. 2000; Pittschieler et al. 2008; Pang 2019).

6.2.2 Potential Harms of Folic Acid Supplementation During Pregnancy in Women with Epilepsy

Congenital malformations (CMs) are recognized as one of the major problems in the field of maternal and child health in both developed and developing countries. In recent years, there have been many studies on the effects of folic acid on pregnancy outcomes, but there are few studies on the optimal recommended dose of folic acid for women of childbearing age. There is no unified standard. In addition, taking folic acid during pregnancy is not absolutely safe. When taking WWE supplements, you need to be aware of the interaction between folic acid and ASMs, and studies have shown that high doses of folic acid can also cause adverse effects on pregnancy and offspring. A randomized controlled trial of different doses of folic acid supplements in pregnant women with epilepsy could be promising for determining the optimal dose in clinical practice.

6.2.3 Interactions Between Folic Acid and Antiseizure Medications

Numerous studies on the safety of folic acid use in women with epilepsy have concluded that taking certain ASMs (including PHT, PB, and CBZ) while taking folic acid may lead to an increase in seizures, possibly due to interactions between the two that accelerate drug metabolism and thus reduce ASM concentrations in plasma. The instructions for the use of folic acid emphasize that large doses of folic acid can antagonize the anti-epileptic effects of PB, PHT, and primidone, so the dosage of folic acid in patients taking these drugs should not exceed 1 mg/day, and no less than 0.4 mg is appropriate.

Many previous studies on the effects of folic acid on the steady-state pharmacokinetics of phenytoin have shown that folic acid can lead to an increase in the oxidative metabolism of phenytoin. One study found that in male patients with epilepsy who took 1 mg/day oral folic acid alongside phenytoin sodium, the serum total phenytoin concentration decreased by 22.6–13.0% on average. There was also a case report of a patient with epilepsy who was treated with 300 mg/day of phenytoin sodium orally for 3 years without seizures, but 1 day after adding 5 mg/day of folic acid to treat macrocytic anemia, their serum phenytoin levels decreased significantly and the patient developed generalized tonic-clonic seizures again. The above-noted correlation between folic acid and phenytoin metabolism suggests that folic acid is a co-factor of phenytoin metabolism, and higher levels of folic acid may increase the affinity of metabolic enzymes, thus greatly improving the efficiency of phenytoin degradation. In addition, there have been case reports of reduced serum levels of carbamazepine and phenobarbital with folic acid administration. Recent molecular docking studies reported potential interactions between ASMs and folic acid in transporters of placenta (Sha et al. 2023) (Fig. 6.1). However, there is a lack of research evidence on the interaction between folic acid and ASMs.

6.2.4 Other Potential Adverse Risks of Folic Acid Supplementation During Pregnancy

It is advocated that WWE supplement folic acid during pregnancy to reduce the occurrence of adverse pregnancy outcomes in offspring, especially for patients who continue to take ASMs during pregnancy. However, folic acid supplementation during pregnancy also carries a number of potential adverse risks for WWE. In addition to potential drug–drug interactions within the mother, folic acid may also directly

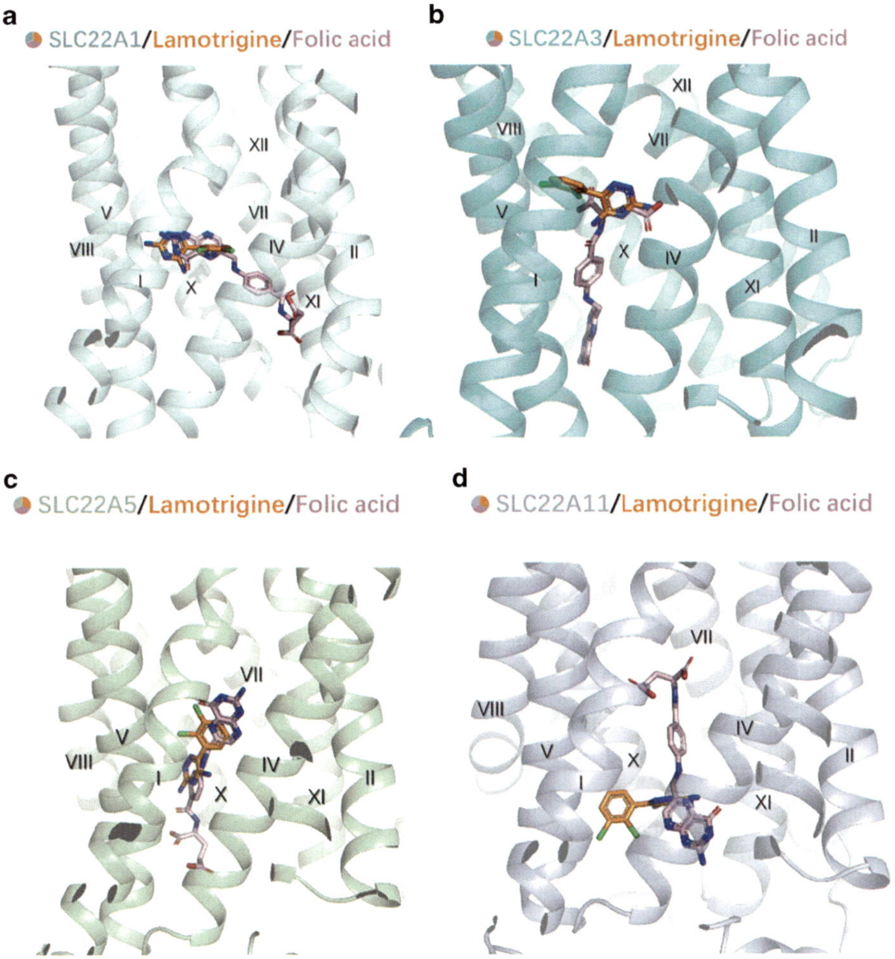

Fig. 6.1 Binding model of folic acid (pink) with receptors. SLC22A1 (**a**), SLC22A3 (**b**), SLC22A5 (**c**), and SLC22A11 (**d**) bind folic acid in a similar manner to lamotrigine, and when transported at the same time, folic acid may compete with lamotrigine

affect fetal brain development. Under normal circumstances, the placenta concentrates folic acid into the fetal circulation, so the level of folic acid in the fetus is 2–4 times higher than that of the mother, and this nutrient is needed for rapid fetal growth and cell proliferation. A recent animal study in which rats were given large doses of folic acid before and during pregnancy found that their offspring had a 42% reduction in IQ, leading to the inference that high levels of folic acid during pregnancy may have an adverse effect on fetal brain development.

High doses of folic acid may lead to an increase in the frequency of seizures. Other animal studies have shown that high doses of folic acid administered to mice before and during pregnancy can reduce the seizure threshold of offspring by 42%. The mechanism of this may be related to the fact that high doses of folic acid changes the stability of the offspring's brain network and increases neuronal excitability, thus reducing the offspring's seizure threshold.

In addition, studies have shown that high levels of folic acid can increase the level of cell methylation, leading to the growth of cancer cells. A nationwide observational cohort study conducted in Denmark, Norway, and Sweden from 1997 to 2017 looked at the effects of mothers with epilepsy and high doses of folic acid taken during pregnancy on childhood cancer risk, observing an increased risk of cancer in children born to mothers with epilepsy. However, the difference between an intake of more than 4 mg of folic acid per day and an intake of less than 3 mg/day was not significant, so there is no valid evidence for a relationship between prenatal exposure to high doses of folic acid and the risk of cancer in children of mothers with epilepsy.

References

Adab N, Kini U, Vinten J, et al. The longer term outcome of children born to mothers with epilepsy. J Neurol Neurosurg Psychiatry. 2004;75(11):1575–83.

Hernandez Diaz S, Werler MM, Walker AM, et al. Folic acid antagonists during pregnancy and the risk of birth defects. N Engl J Med. 2000;343(22):1608–14.

Meador KJ, Pennell PB, May RC, et al. Effects of periconceptional folate on cognition in children of women with epilepsy: NEAD study. Neurology. 2020;94(7):e729–40.

Pang J. Effect of folic acid on pregnancy complications and pregnancy outcome in female epileptic patients treated with antiepileptic drugs. Tianjin Medical University; 2019.

Pittschieler S, Brezinka C, Jahn B, et al. Spontaneous abortion and the prophylactic effect of folic acid supplementation in epileptic women undergoing antiepileptic therapy. J Neurol. 2008;255(12):1926–31.

Sha L, Yong X, Shao Z, Duan Y, Hong Q, Zhang J, Zhang Y, Chen L. Targeting adverse effects of antiseizure medication on offspring: current evidence and new strategies for safety. Expert Rev Neurother. 2023;23(2):141–56. https://doi.org/10.1080/14737175.2023.2176751. Epub 2023 Feb 12.

Suggested Readings

Breen DP, Davenport RJ. Teratogenicity of antiepileptic drugs. BMJ. 2006;333(7569):615–6.

Chitayat D, Matsui D, Amitai Y, et al. Folic acid supplementation for pregnant women and those planning pregnancy: 2015 update. J Clin Pharmacol. 2016;56(2):170–5.

Crawford P. Best practice guidelines for the management of women with epilepsy. Epilepsia. 2005;46:117–24.

Electroencephalogram and Epilepsy Group of the Chinese Society of Nerurology. Guidelines for the management of peri-pregnant women with epilepsy in China. Chin J Neurol. 2021;54(6):539–44.

Epilepsy in pregnancy, in RCOG green-top guideline No. 68. 2016.

Girotto F, Scott L, Avchalumov Y, et al. High dose folic acid supplementation of rats alters synaptic transmission and seizure susceptibility in offspring. Sci Rep. 2013;3:1465.

Greene ND, Stanier P, Moore GE. The emerging role of epigenetic mechanisms in the etiology of neural tube defects. Epigenetics. 2011;6(7):875–83.

Kjaer D, Horvath-Puho E, Christensen J, et al. Antiepileptic drug use, folic acid supplementation, and congenital abnormalities: a population-based case-control study. BJOG. 2008;115(1):98–103.

Morrow JI, Hunt SJ, Russell AJ, et al. Folic acid use and major congenital malformations in offspring of women with epilepsy: a prospective study from the UK Epilepsy and Pregnancy Register. J Neurol Neurosurg Psychiatry. 2009;80(5):506–11.

Pickell L, Brown K, Li D, et al. High intake of folic acid disrupts embryonic development in mice. Birth Defects Res A Clin Mol Teratol. 2011;91(1):8–19.

Steinweg DL, Bentley ML. Seizures following reduction in phenytoin level after orally administered folic acid. Neurology. 2005;64(11):1982.

Taylor CM, Atkinson C, Penfold C, et al. Folic acid in pregnancy and 22 mortality from cancer and cardiovascular disease: further follow-up of the Aberdeen folic acid supplementation trial. J Epidemiol Community Health. 2015;69(8):789–94.

Tomson T, Battino D, Bonizzoni E, et al. Dose-dependent risk of malformations with antiepileptic drugs: an analysis of data from the EURAP epilepsy and pregnancy registry. Lancet Neurol. 2011;10(7):609–17.

Tomson T, Sha L, Chen L. Management of epilepsy in pregnancy: what we still need to learn. Epilepsy Behav Rep. 2023;24:100624. https://doi.org/10.1016/j.ebr.2023.100624.

7 Postpartum Management for Women with Epilepsy

Tianhong Zhang, Ziyi Chen, and Yifei Duan

7.1 Postpartum Complications

Tianhong Zhang

Peripartum depression is prevalent and impacts childbearing, with substantial adverse effects on both pregnancy outcomes and the developing child. These conditions encompass major and minor depressive episodes occurring during pregnancy or within the initial 12 months following delivery. While sharing similarities with depressive episodes occurring outside the peripartum period, they maintain distinct diagnostic criteria.

Individuals with epilepsy face a heightened susceptibility to experiencing depression, as highlighted in previous studies (Rai et al. 2012). The prevalence of mood disorders in adult epilepsy cohorts varies between 10% and 50%, depending on prevalence estimates and whether the study samples are drawn from epilepsy centers or the general population. These conditions stand out as robust predictors of the quality of life in individuals with epilepsy. Furthermore, they are closely associated with challenges such as suboptimal seizure control, adverse effects of antiseizure medications, cognitive difficulties, thoughts of self-harm, and result in substantial economic burdens on society.

T. Zhang (✉)
Shanghai Mental Health Center, Shanghai Jiaotong University School of Medicine, Shanghai, China

Z. Chen
Department of Neurology, The First Affiliated Hospital, Sun Yat-sen University, Guangzhou, China
e-mail: chenziyi@mail.sysu.edu.cn

Y. Duan
Department of Neurology, West China Hospital, Sichuan University, Chengdu, China

L. Chen (ed.), *Women with Epilepsy in Child-bearing Age*,
https://doi.org/10.1007/978-981-97-3921-9_7

The psychiatric aspects of epilepsy during pregnancy have often been overlooked. The focus on preventing epileptic seizures and the potential teratogenic effects of antiepileptic medications has tended to overshadow considerations of depressive symptoms. Nevertheless, it is crucial to recognize that maternal psychological well-being plays a pivotal role in ensuring the mother's self-care and the well-being of her children. Consequently, healthcare providers should be well-informed about the prevalence, indicators, ramifications, and available interventions for psychiatric disorders in pregnant individuals with epilepsy.

7.1.1 The Frequency for Postpartum Depression in Women with Epilepsy

Pregnancy and the postpartum phase can represent critical periods characterized by an elevated risk of major depressive episodes, and this vulnerability may be heightened in women with epilepsy. In the broader population, the occurrence of depressive episodes affects as many as 13% of pregnant women. During the postpartum period, this rate escalates to approximately 19% according to findings from certain studies (Bennett et al. 2004; Gavin et al. 2005).

In two separate studies, Turner et al. discovered that the point prevalence of postpartum depression 5–8 weeks after childbirth was over three times greater in women who had recently given birth compared to their healthy counterparts. In an initial investigation involving 35 women with epilepsy alongside 35 matched controls, the findings revealed a higher incidence of postpartum depression among women with epilepsy (29%) compared to those without epilepsy (11%), as assessed using the Edinburgh Postnatal Depression Scale. Subsequently, the same research group conducted a follow-up study involving 55 women with epilepsy and control participants, revealing that 39% of women with epilepsy experienced postpartum depression in contrast to 12% of the control group. These studies, however, did not establish any discernible links between the severity of postpartum depressive symptoms and factors such as epilepsy type, seizure frequency, or the choice between monotherapy and polytherapy antiseizure medication regimens (Turner et al. 2006, 2009; Galanti et al. 2009).

In contrast, another study involving 56 women with epilepsy found that 25% exhibited elevated Beck Depression Inventory scores during the postpartum period, with these scores being associated with antiseizure medication polytherapy and postpartum seizures.

Drawing on data from the Norwegian Mother and Child Cohort Study, which encompassed 329 women with epilepsy and 106,224 pregnancies in individuals without epilepsy, symptoms of depression during pregnancy were more prevalent in women with epilepsy (19%) relative to the comparison group (11%), as assessed using the Hopkins Symptom Checklist in the second trimester (Reiter et al. 2013). Further analyses within this cohort, conducted over an extended period with multiple assessment points, underscored elevated rates of depression and anxiety during both pregnancy and the postpartum phase. The analyses indicated that women with epilepsy exhibited higher rates of depression (26.7%) during pregnancy compared to individuals without epilepsy (18.9%). This trend persisted at various time points, with point prevalence rates consistently higher. Notably, a significantly smaller proportion of depressed women with epilepsy used antidepressive medication during pregnancy compared to women without epilepsy and women with other chronic conditions (4.6% vs. 13.2% and 15.5%, respectively). This difference in medication use could be attributed to efforts to reduce overall drug exposure during pregnancy, although it is important to mention that even women with epilepsy who did not use antiseizure medications during pregnancy had a low frequency of antidepressant use (2.6%). Consequently, the lower utilization of antidepressants among women with epilepsy could not be solely attributed to concurrent antiseizure medications.

Overall, research has highlighted the increased vulnerability of women with epilepsy to experience postpartum depression and anxiety during pregnancy and the postpartum period. Multiple studies have consistently shown higher rates of these psychiatric symptoms in women with epilepsy compared to women without epilepsy. However, the specific factors contributing to these elevated rates, such as epilepsy type, seizure frequency, and medication regimens, remain complex and not fully understood. Recognizing and addressing the psychological well-being of women with epilepsy during pregnancy and the postpartum period is essential to ensure optimal maternal care and, by extension, the well-being of their children.

7.1.2 The Risk Factors for Postpartum Depression in Women with Epilepsy

Women with epilepsy face specific risk factors that can contribute to the development of peripartum depression, which are critical to understand and address for better maternal mental health. Several prominent risk factors within the epilepsy cohort have been identified in the context of peripartum depression:

1. High seizure frequency: Women with epilepsy and frequent seizures are at an elevated risk for peripartum depression. The constant threat and unpredictability of seizures can contribute to heightened stress and emotional distress during pregnancy and the postpartum period.
2. Adverse socioeconomic factors: Socioeconomic challenges, such as financial stress, limited access to healthcare, or inadequate social support, can significantly increase the risk of peripartum depression in women with epilepsy.
3. History of physical and/or sexual abuse: Women who have experienced physical or sexual abuse in their past may have a higher vulnerability to peripartum depression, as such traumatic experiences can resurface or intensify during pregnancy.
4. Previous loss of a child: Women who have previously suffered the loss of a child, whether due to epilepsy-related complications or other reasons, may experience heightened depression during subsequent pregnancies.

5. Unplanned pregnancy: Unplanned pregnancies can be emotionally challenging for anyone but can be particularly distressing for women with epilepsy who may not have had the opportunity to adequately plan for managing their epilepsy and mental health during pregnancy.
6. Prepregnancy depression: A history of depression prior to pregnancy is a well-established risk factor for peripartum depression in women with epilepsy. These preexisting mental health conditions can be exacerbated during pregnancy.

The following studies have identified these risk factors:

According to findings by Galanti et al. (2009), certain factors are linked to postpartum depression among women with epilepsy. Specifically, antiseizure medication polytherapy, having multiple children (multiparity), and experiencing tonic-clonic seizures during the postpartum period were all associated with an increased risk of depression. Notably, the use of lamotrigine, a commonly prescribed antiseizure medication, did not demonstrate a reduced risk compared to other antiseizure medications. Surprisingly, depression rates appeared to be higher in groups of women with epilepsy treated with lamotrigine, irrespective of their previous episodes of major depression. Consequently, the authors concluded that mood-stabilizing antiseizure medications did not appear to mitigate the risk of postnatal depression in women with epilepsy.

Bjork et al. (2015) revealed that the risk of experiencing peripartum depression was most pronounced in patients who used antiseizure medications, particularly those receiving polytherapy. Additionally, patients administered higher antiseizure medication doses and/or possessing elevated plasma concentrations were at greater risk compared to individuals with lower doses and concentrations. Notably, no specific antiseizure medication demonstrated a risk-reducing effect. Within a subgroup characterized by high seizure frequency during pregnancy, the risk of peripartum depression was particularly elevated. Long-term outcomes were less favorable for women with epilepsy who had a history of depression or had experienced previous instances of sexual or physical abuse. However, prognosis was generally comparable between different groups of women with epilepsy. Interestingly, for women with epilepsy, peripartum depressive symptoms were less likely to represent the first episode of depression. The study also indicated that the association between peripartum depression and psychosocial risk factors exhibited similarities across women with epilepsy, women without epilepsy, and women with other chronic diseases. This suggests that certain psychosocial factors may have comparable effects on peripartum mental health in diverse populations, underscoring the importance of recognizing and addressing these factors through healthcare interventions.

As mentioned previously, the incidence and prevalence of peripartum depression are notably elevated within specific subgroups of women, particularly those using antiseizure medications. Antiseizure medications have garnered attention for their potential negative psychotropic effects, a concern that gained prominence after the U.S. Food and Drug Administration (FDA) issued a warning in 2008 regarding the risk of suicidal thoughts and behavior in antiseizure medication-treated patients. Nevertheless, it is essential to acknowledge that antiseizure medication use during pregnancy is closely intertwined with epilepsy activity and its severity. Unmedicated patients rarely experienced seizures during the 2 years before or during pregnancy. Given this strong association between antiseizure medication use and seizure activity, it is challenging to disentangle the effects of these factors in relation to the risk of depression.

Bjork et al. also unveiled a bidirectional relationship between epilepsy severity, uncontrolled epilepsy, and psychiatric disorders, corroborating findings from other studies. Notably, patients with multiple seizures during pregnancy were the group most frequently affected by depression. The psychological burden associated with frequent seizures during pregnancy may contribute to an exacerbation of depressive symptoms. Additionally, a history of previous depression was associated with a higher likelihood of experiencing frequent epileptic seizures during pregnancy. This suggests that preexisting psychiatric conditions may serve as markers not only for an increased risk of peripartum depression but also for heightened seizure activity during pregnancy. These findings align with research in nonpregnant patients, highlighting a connection between seizure frequency and depression. Various mechanisms may underlie this co-occurrence, with neurobiological processes related to seizure development potentially inducing psychiatric symptoms.

Recognizing these risk factors is crucial for healthcare providers to provide targeted support and interventions for women with epilepsy during pregnancy and the postpartum period. Comprehensive care should include regular mental health assessments, individualized treatment plans, and access to support networks to help women with epilepsy manage their epilepsy and maintain optimal mental well-being during this critical time.

7.1.3 The Neurobiological and Psychological Mechanisms for Postpartum Depression in Women with Epilepsy

The co-occurrence of peripartum depression and epilepsy in women with epilepsy is a complex phenomenon with multiple underlying mechanisms, including both neurobiological and psychological factors (Fig. 7.1).

Neurobiological mechanisms:

1. Seizure-induced neurobiological changes: The neurobiological processes associated with the development of seizures can potentially induce psychiatric symptoms. Seizures are known to disrupt normal brain functioning and the postictal state, characterized by altered consciousness and cognitive impairment, may contribute to mood disturbances.
2. Frontal and temporal hypofunction: Electrophysiologic and neuroimaging studies have implicated frontal and temporal hypofunction in women with epilepsy. These regions of the brain are involved in mood regulation and dysfunction in these areas can lead to emotional instability and depressive symptoms.
3. Serotonergic and glutaminergic dysfunction: Dysregulation of neurotransmitter systems, such as serotonin and glutamate, has been observed in epilepsy. These neurotransmitters play a crucial role in mood regulation and their dysfunction can contribute to the development of depressive symptoms.

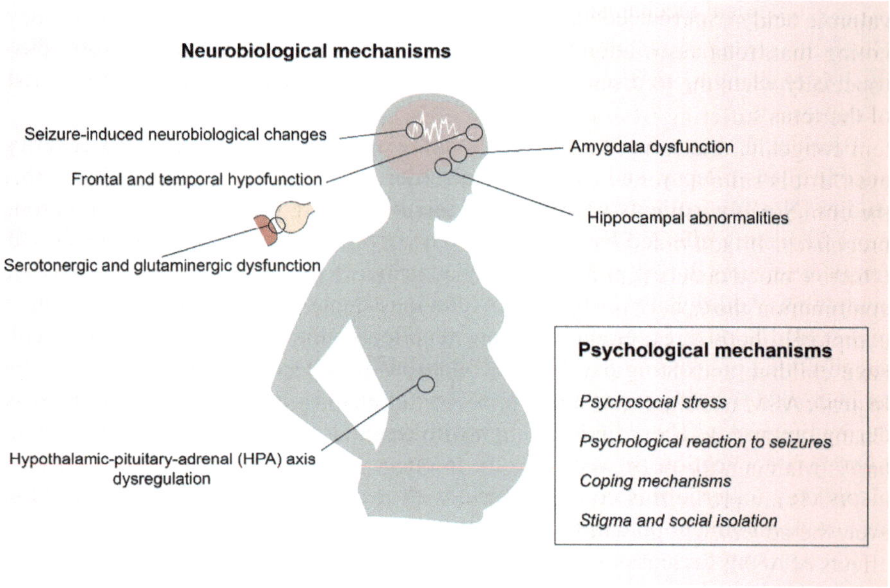

Fig. 7.1 Neurobiological and psychological mechanisms for postpartum depression in women with epilepsy

4. Hypothalamic-pituitary-adrenal (HPA) axis dysregulation: The HPA axis is a key component in the body's stress response. Dysregulation of the HPA axis, characterized by abnormal cortisol levels, has been associated with both epilepsy and depression. Altered cortisol levels can influence mood and contribute to depressive symptoms.
5. Amygdala dysfunction: The amygdala, a brain region involved in processing emotions, has been implicated in the association between depression and epilepsy. Dysfunctional amygdala activity may contribute to the development of anxiety and mood disorders in women with epilepsy.
6. Hippocampal abnormalities: In an early study conducted by Quiske et al. (2000), it was observed that individuals with hippocampal sclerosis had higher scores on the Beck Depression Inventory (BDI) compared to those with temporal lobe epilepsy but no hippocampal abnormalities. However, it is worth noting that the mean BDI scores in the group with hippocampal sclerosis fell within the range indicating mild depression. This finding was subsequently replicated in another study, where hippocampal atrophy was specifically linked to the contralateral hemisphere of seizure onset. A later study, which involved the diagnosis of depression based on the Structured Clinical Inventory for DSM-IV (SCID), also found an association between hippocampal atrophy and depression. However, it is important to acknowledge that not all studies have identified a significant association between hippocampal abnormalities and depression in patients with epilepsy.

Psychological mechanisms:

1. Psychosocial stress: The challenges associated with living with epilepsy, including the fear of seizures, stigma, and limitations on daily activities, can lead to chronic stress. Chronic stress is a known risk factor for the development of depression.
2. Psychological reaction to seizures: Experiencing seizures can be psychologically distressing. The unpredictability and potential loss of control during a seizure can lead to feelings of anxiety and depression.
3. Coping mechanisms: Coping with the demands of epilepsy management, medication side effects, and the added stressors of pregnancy and motherhood can strain coping mechanisms. Ineffective coping strategies may contribute to the development of peripartum depression.
4. Stigma and social isolation: Stigma related to epilepsy can lead to social isolation and feelings of loneliness, which are risk factors for depression. The perception of being misunderstood or judged by others can exacerbate emotional distress.

In summary, the co-occurrence of peripartum depression and epilepsy in women with epilepsy involves a complex interplay of neurobiological and psychological factors. Understanding these mechanisms is crucial for providing comprehensive care and support to women with epilepsy during pregnancy and the postpartum period, as it allows for targeted interventions to mitigate the risk and impact of peripartum depression.

7.1.4 Recommendations for the Management of Postpartum Depression in Women with Epilepsy

Recommendations for Antidepressant Use

A review focused on the treatment of moderate postnatal depression in women without epilepsy and found that selective serotonin reuptake inhibitors (SSRIs) were more effective than placebo in terms of response and remission rates. While there is a paucity of methodologically rigorous studies evaluating the efficacy of antidepressant treatment in epilepsy, it is generally assumed that depressive symptoms in individuals with epilepsy, outside of pregnancy, tend to respond well to SSRIs and certain serotonin-norepinephrine reuptake inhibitors (SNRIs) (Lin et al. 2012). It is rare to observe an exacerbation of seizures upon initiating SSRI treatment (Lin et al. 2012). In cases where patients are already receiving antiseizure medications, medications such as citalopram, escitalopram, and venlafaxine are considered favorable options due to their minimal interference with the cytochrome P450 (CYP) enzymes. Conversely, CYP inducers like carbamazepine and phenytoin may reduce the serum levels of most SSRIs and SNRIs, while CYP inhibitors like valproate can increase their concentrations.

Extensive research has been conducted to assess the risks of adverse events associated with antidepressant use during pregnancy. The SSRIs are known to pass through the placenta in substantial quantities, are considered to be relatively safe, and have seen widespread use in pregnancy in recent years. There is concern that exposure to these medications in utero may lead to adverse effects in offspring, including the potential for cardiac defects, respiratory distress, and low birth weight. However, research findings have been conflicting, likely due to the various confounding factors associated with maternal psychiatric conditions.

Numerous clinical studies based on registries, along with preclinical data, have indicated a low but notable risk of persistent pulmonary hypertension, as well as an elevated risk of transient disturbances in sleep patterns and temporary neonatal jitteriness and irritability following in utero exposure to these medications. Concerning the long-term effects on offspring, some studies have suggested an increased risk of cognitive, behavioral, and developmental problems, even after accounting for maternal mood disorders.

A review article recommended non-pharmacological treatments as the first-line therapy during pregnancy. However, it is important to acknowledge that non-pharmacological options may not always be feasible or effective. Balancing the potential teratogenic risks of SSRIs with the potentially severe consequences of maternal depression is crucial when determining the most appropriate course of treatment during pregnancy.

In women with epilepsy, individualized cost-benefit assessments are particularly important. This is because there are a lack of data regarding the consequences of combining antiseizure medications with SSRIs during pregnancy. The decision to initiate effective, rapid-onset therapies must carefully consider the potential risks and benefits in the context of women with epilepsy, where seizure control and maternal well-being are paramount concerns.

Recommendations for Antiseizure Medication Use

Several studies have reported an association between antiseizure medication therapy and peripartum depression in women with epilepsy, with three studies highlighting this connection. Interestingly, antiseizure medication considered to be "mood stabilizing" did not appear to reduce the risk of peripartum depression. It is worth noting that the co-occurrence of psychiatric and psychotropic properties in antiseizure medication prescriptions could potentially introduce selection bias. However, these findings remained consistent even after accounting for a previous history of psychiatric disorders. Furthermore, it is challenging to fully disentangle the relationship between antiseizure medication therapy and the severity of epilepsy, as evidenced by the strong link between seizure frequency and peripartum psychiatric symptoms.

Regarding side effects, the same antiseizure medication may have both positive and negative psychotropic effects. Antiseizure medications like carbamazepine, valproate, oxcarbazepine, lamotrigine, and pregabalin are believed to have positive effects on mood, while phenobarbital, phenytoin, vigabatrin, levetiracetam, topiramate, tiagabine, zonisamide, and felbamate are suspected to negatively impact mood.

Anxiety can also emerge after discontinuing an antiseizure medication with anxiolytic properties. However, it is important to note that observed positive mood effects related to anticonvulsant treatment in women with epilepsy do not necessarily imply therapeutic efficacy for depression or anxiety disorders in individuals without epilepsy. Robust evidence supporting the positive effects of antiseizure medications on psychiatric disorders only exists in trials involving patients with psychiatric conditions but without epilepsy. In epilepsy, the underlying etiology and the spectrum of mood disorder symptoms can differ from other populations, and complicating factors such as antiseizure medication polytherapy and cognitive dysfunction are often present. While add-on therapy with antiseizure medications that have positive psychotropic effects has been suggested to have some impact on psychiatric symptoms in a recent review, it does not appear to be more effective than treatment with antidepressant medication or psychotherapy. Due to the negative associations between polytherapy and depression, it is not recommended to treat depression or anxiety related to pregnancy by adding antiseizure medications to the treatment regimen. And the possible interactions between antiseizure medications and antidepressants should be considered when treating peripatum depression in women with epilepsy.

Recommendations for Childcare

When caring for an infant, individuals with epilepsy often grapple with the unpredictability of seizures, which can give rise to a profound sense of vulnerability and fear of inadvertently causing harm to their child. These fears may encompass concerns such as the possibility of dropping the child during myoclonic jerks or tonic-clonic seizures, or leaving the child unattended during a generalized seizure or in the postictal period. In a survey focused on childcare issues among mothers with epilepsy, activities like going outdoors and bathing the child were rated as particularly challenging. These apprehensions are not unwarranted, as evidenced by a study involving 28 mothers with severe epilepsy who had not received childcare guidance before childbirth. Tragic events resulting from maternal seizures have been shown to affect 32% of their offspring during the first year of life, including two near-drowning accidents and six instances of dropping the child, one of which was fatal. Inappropriate handling of the child during non-convulsive seizures was also observed. Importantly, the majority of these incidents could have been prevented. In contrast, a control group of mothers with epilepsy who had received guidance on safe childcare experienced very few unfortunate events.

To mitigate unnecessary anxiety, it is crucial that parents with epilepsy who are expecting a child receive advice on safe childcare practices. They should be reassured that, by following guidelines, the likelihood of harm to their child due to parental seizures is minimal. This information should also be conveyed to individuals with well-controlled epilepsy, particularly during the postpartum period when there is a potential for seizure recurrence and myoclonic jerks. As adhering to safety recommendations often necessitates the presence of another person, single mothers with epilepsy can be especially susceptible to anxiety related to childcare. Given the prevalence of single motherhood within epilepsy populations, it is essential to provide additional support to these women.

7.2 Breastfeeding in Women with Epilepsy

Yifei Duan

7.2.1 Safety of Breastfeeding for Women with Epilepsy

The safety of breastfeeding while taking antiepileptic medications is a major concern for many women with epilepsy, and fewer WWE choose to breastfeed than women without epilepsy. However, ASM use is not contraindicated while breastfeeding, and current national and international guidelines advocate breastfeeding for women with epilepsy. Studies have shown that although fat-soluble antiepileptic drugs are present in WWE breast milk, in most cases it is difficult for the ASMs to penetrate the breast milk barrier, making the ASM content in breast milk insufficient to have adverse effects. At the same time, previous studies that measured the blood levels of ASMs in postpartum mothers and breastfed infants who were exposed to ASMs showed that the blood levels of infants were much lower than those of mothers, and below the lower limit of the reference range. In addition, mothers who take ASMs and insist on breastfeeding do not affect their children's near- or long-term psychomotor development. Therefore, when WWE receive postpartum counseling, clinicians should inform them that it is a well-established fact that breastfeeding has great benefits for the baby and that it is generally safe for women who take ASMs to breastfeed.

Previous studies have also shown that breast milk may have higher concentrations of barbiturates, benzodiazepines, lamotrigine, zonisamide and ethosuximide, which can lead to adverse effects (such as drowsiness and irritability), so it is important for WWE taking these drugs to monitor offspring for adverse effects during feeding. The relative infant dose (RID) is an important measure for evaluating the risk of lactation with a drug, and a RID below 10 is considered safe. Of the available ASMs in the country, only phenobarbital and topiramate have a RID of more than 10 (24 and 24.5, respectively). In summary, we recommend that WWE should avoid medications such as phenobarbital, benzodiazepines, and topiramate when breastfeeding, and that newborns should be closely monitored for ASM-related adverse reactions (such as drowsiness, difficulty breastfeeding, excessive irritability and crying, and skin rash) when their breastfeeding mothers take ASMs. Breastfeeding should be suspended if any concerns exist.

7.2.2 Considerations for Breastfeeding

WWE should pay attention to posture when breastfeeding; wraparound and lie feeding are more appropriate breastfeeding positions for WWE, as lying feeding is most likely to reduce the likelihood of an accidental fall injury to the baby. During the feeding process, the family should pay attention at all times and, if the patient has seizures, the baby's mouth and nose should be checked to ensure they are not blocked and causing suffocation. In addition, sitting is also a relatively safe posture, and when sitting the mother should try to ensure that the surrounding area is flat and soft, so as to avoid an accidental fall of the baby onto a hard surface.

In addition, the timing of breastfeeding needs to be duly considered. Usually the newborn receives day and night feeding 7–8 times, with lactation periods approximately 3 h apart; this reduces to 6–7 times a day after 2 weeks, 6 times a day after 2–3 months, 5–6 times a day at 4–5 months. Frequent breastfeeding makes the mother easy to tire, especially with night feeding, and lack of sleep as well as poor rest can induce seizures.

In order to prevent seizures, it is recommended that patients should let the baby eat enough during the day, ensure the baby's adequate intake during the day, feed on demand at night, ensure the quality of a baby's sleep, but also ensure that it is conducive to the patient's own sleep requirements. At the same time, the mother should learn to lie feed, as lie feeding can greatly alleviate the patient's body load bearing, and can also allow the mother to rest while nursing.

7.3 Effects of Antiseizure Medications on Offspring

Yifei Duan

In addition to obstetric risks, WWE face a higher risk of adverse outcomes for their offspring. Women with epilepsy tend to be concerned about the negative effects of seizures, comorbidities, and exposure of ASMs on the fetus. To date, only a few commonly used ASMs have been systematically investigated to understand the associated risks of malformation and neurodevelopment, and the safety of most ASMs in this regard remains unclear. The number of people enrolled in the newer ASM teratogenicity pregnancy registry is still smaller than the number of traditional ASMs, and there is still no valid evidence regarding teratogenicity for many of the newer ASMs. As prescription of ASMs with relatively unclear evidence are becoming more and more prevalent in pregnant women with epilepsy, it is essential to provide safety evidence for those ASMs. With cohort data accumulating, potential teratogenicity of such ASMs may be referred to safety data in adult patients with epilepsy. For example, if a certain ASM is observed a hepatic toxic effect in adult patients with epilepsy, it could be associated with teratogenicity of the same organ in fetus of pregnant women with epilepsy exposed to the ASM. However, this hypothesis is lacking evidence.

7.3.1 Effects of Antiseizure Medications on the Fetus

The treatment of patients with epilepsy mainly relies on the use of ASMs. ASMs are prescribed to reduce the severity of epilepsy during pregnancy, however, the adverse reactions of ASMs on the fetus of women with epilepsy cannot be ignored. The effects of ASMs on embryos or fetuses are mainly manifested in the following three aspects: (1) major congenital malformations (MCMs), (2) neurodevelopmental disorders, (3) fetal anticonvulsant syndromes, and (4) intrauterine growth restrictions. The above effects will increase the needs of patients' families for medical or educational intervention as well as the socioeconomic burden.

The effects of antiseizure medications on the fetus are mainly manifested in the teratogenicity of ASMs. Previous studies have shown that when embryos are exposed to ASMs, the probability of MCMs is 4–9%, which is 2–3 times higher than that of the general population. Figure 7.2 showed the Classic MCMs caused by valproic acid and carbamazepine.

Current studies consistently show that the second-generation ASMs LTG and LEV are significantly superior to traditional ASMs such as VPA, CBZ, and PHT in terms of drug safety, teratogenicity, and impact on the neurodevelopment of offspring. Therefore, it is recommended that ASMs such as LTG or LEV should be used whenever possible in pregnant WWE to benefit the health of their offspring.

The teratogenicity of some ASMs has been effectively proven by many pregnancy registry studies, prospective cohort studies, and studies based on electronic databases. Tomson et al. classified the teratogenic risk of ASMs with reasonable data, defining low risk to include LTG, LEV, OXC, CBZ, and GBP; medium risk to include PB, TPM, and PHT; and high risk including only VPA. As for the type of malformations, cardiac malformations are the commonest major congenital malformations encountered following exposure to ASMs in utero, while others include neural tube defects, cleft lip and palate, hypospadias, and skeletal malformations. The descriptive results of this review essentially support this conclusion.

Current research has resulted in contradictory conclusions regarding the teratogenic risk of ASM polytherapy; some authors believe that the risk of ASM polytherapy is higher than that of monotherapy, while some think that there is no difference between the two regimens. Frank JE Vajda et al. analyzed the APR data and found that teratogenicity associated with ASM polytherapy may depend more on the use of VPA or TPM; that is, the teratogenicity risk of ASMs that combine with either VPA or TPM is significantly higher than combinations involving other ASMs. In contrast to VPA and TPM, the use of CBZ, LTG, or LEV in combination with ASMs other than VPA or TPM does not appear to increase teratogenic risk. Notably, Frank JE Vajda et al. also found that for a given dose of VPA, the risk of teratogenicity when VPA was used in combination with other ASMs (such as LTG) was significantly lower than for the same dose of VPA used as monotherapy. This may be caused by increased VPA clearance resulting from the combination of drugs.

Minor congenital malformations usually require very careful examination and long-term follow-up, so they are often difficult to evaluate in clinical studies. About 6–20% of the offspring of women with epilepsy were found to have minor congenital malformations, about twice the rate of the general population, which may be related to later cognitive development disorders.

The risk of ASM teratogenicity is associated with the type of drug, the dose, and the presence or absence of multidrug therapy (Table 7.1). The results of a British epilepsy pregnancy registry study show that the overall incidence of MCMs in

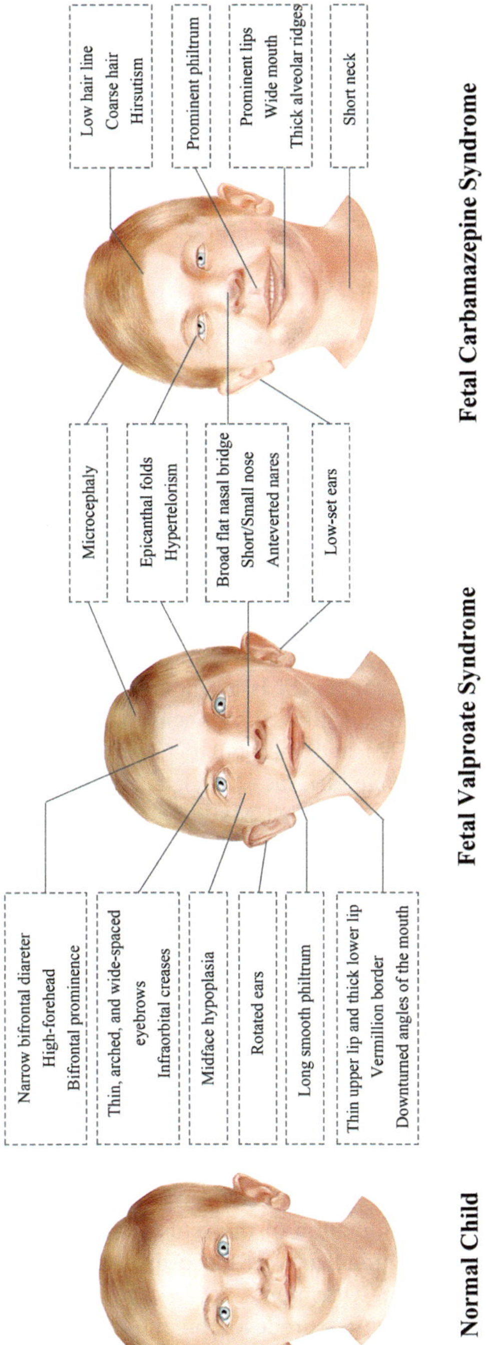

Fig. 7.2 Classic MCMs caused by valproic acid and carbamazepine

Table 7.1 Teratogenicity of common antiseizure medications

Drugs	Teratogenic types	Effects	Embryo-fetal risk
VPA	Neural tube malformations, cleft lip and palate, heart abnormalities, developmental delays	10% for single drugs, higher for multiple drugs	There are
PTH	Fetal hydantoin syndrome: Craniofacial malformations, hypoplastic nails, fetal growth restriction, heart abnormalities, cleft lip, and palate	5–11%	There are
CBZ, OXC	Spina bifida	1–2%	There are
PB	Cleft lip and palate, heart abnormalities, urinary tract malformations	10–12%	Possible
LGT	Cleft lip and palate	Less than 1%	Possible
TPM	Cleft lip and palate	2–3%	Possible
LEV	Abnormal bones, abnormal growth	Primary observations	Possibly

fetuses exposed to ASMs during pregnancy in women with epilepsy is only 4.2%, slightly higher than that of pregnant women with epilepsy who does not take ASMs (3.5%), but the teratogenic rate can be as high as 17%, and the teratogenic risk will be further increased if valproic acid is included in the drug regimen. Teratogenicity varies by specific ASM. The latest prospective study by EURAP compared the incidence of MCMs when using eight ASMs as monotherapy, finding valproic acid (10.3%) to have the highest risk, followed by phenobarbital (6.5%) and phenytoin (6.4%). Carbamazepine (5.5%) and topiramate (3.9%) were in the middle-risk group. Oxcarbazepine (3.0%), lamotrigine (2.9%), and levetiracetam (2.8%) showed a higher safety, with the incidence of MCMs in women taking these ASMs being comparable to that of pregnant women with epilepsy who did not take ASMs. Studies of epileptic pregnancy registries in North America and Denmark have also shown significantly higher teratogenicity rates for valproic acid than for other ASMs. In addition, the risk of teratogenicity with ASMs is dose-dependent; when the total daily dose of valproic acid is ≤650 mg, the incidence of MCMs is 6.3%, above which the teratogenicity is significantly increased. The total daily safe dose of carbamazepine and lamotrigine is 700 and 325 mg, respectively, but whether these safe threshold values are appropriate for the East Asian population is unclear.

In addition to the effects of drug type, dose, and combination of drugs, the impact of drug exposure period on the fetus is important. Exposure to ASMs during the first trimester has the greatest impact on the fetus. Weeks 18–20 of gestation is a critical period for the development and formation of embryonic organs, during which a 4-dimensional ultrasound examination of the fetus should be performed to detect possible congenital malformations such as those involving the heart, craniofacial bones, and neural tube in a timely fashion.

As noted above, in the study of neurodevelopmental disorders in offspring, most research has focused on the neurodevelopmental toxicity of VPA. VPA has a wide range of effects on offspring, involving language expression, language comprehension, gross motor skills, attention, memory, executive ability, adaptive ability (especially daily living skills and social skills), and other fields. It can also increase the risk of emotional/behavioral problems, autism spectrum disorders (ASDs), and attention deficit/hyperactivity disorders (ADHD) in offspring. Moreover, its effects have a certain permanence. The effect of VPA on cognitive function in offspring begins at age 3 and continues even up to age 6, when IQ is more stable and strongly correlated with school-age and adult IQ. Intrauterine exposure to VPA is dose-dependent. Taking 800 mg/day as a cut-off threshold, a daily dose of VPA >800 mg in a mother was associated with reduced IQ, verbal skills, non-verbal skills, spatial abilities, memory, and executive function at age 6 in her offspring, and average scores were lower not only than those whose mothers took CBZ, LTG, or in other monotherapy groups, but also lower than those who took these medications in the multitherapy group. Low-dose VPA (<800 mg/day) was only associated with decreased language abilities. Compared with VPA, offspring exposed to LTG or PHT in utero did not show significantly reduced IQ or impaired verbal, non-verbal, and spatial abilities. A study of CBZ found that although CBZ can significantly reduce the language ability of offspring, it has no significant effect on their average IQ. Intrauterine exposure to CBZ may also increase the risk of ADHD in offspring, but the association was not statistically significant. Based on the current clinical data, LTG and LEV are relatively safe ASMs, followed by CBZ and PHT. It is important to note that verbal and non-verbal scores are the same in the normal population, but studies have found that children exposed in utero to the four common ASMs, namely VPA, LTG, PHT, and CBZ, have lower verbal abilities than non-verbal abilities. This difference exists at age 3 and decreases between 3 and 6 years of age. Figure 7.3 demonstrated the neurodevelopmental disorders relating to ASMs from previous published literatures.

7.3.2 Effect of ASMs in Animal Models

Many studies have used animal models to discuss the teratogenic patterns and mechanisms of ASMs, including rodents, primates, and zebrafish. Unlike clinical research conclusions, animal experimental results show that almost all ASMs can cause teratogenic effects, including LTG and LEV, which are relatively safe according to clinical experience. Although these animal models have to some extent reflected the teratogenic patterns of ASMs observed clinically, there are also many issues: the models used are non-epileptic animal models, the doses used do not necessarily have antiepileptic effects, and most studies do not accurately replicate the pattern of 2–3 times daily oral administration of ASMs during pregnancy in women with epilepsy. Animal experiments often use specific time points for drug administration, such as single, multiple, or continuous administration during organ formation, and various methods of administration including oral, subcutaneous injection, intravenous injection, or intraperitoneal injection. In addition to the differences in drug metabolism kinetics among different species, these methods often cannot simulate the fluctuation of drug concentrations in the human body. This can

Assessed domains	VPA	CBZ	PHT	PB	CLN	LTG	LEV	TPM	OXC	PGB
Intellectual/Developmental quotient	34	9	2	2	1	1	0	0	4	
Language	19	1	0	1		1	0			
Learning and Memory	17	1	1	2		2	1	1		
Attention and Executive	9	0	0			0	0			
Motor	6	3	0			2	0			
Social	4	1				0				
Communication	1	1				0				
Emotion	0	1	0	1		0				
Adaptive	4	0	0			0				
Behavior	6	2		1		2	1			
Neurodevelopment disorders	4	2	1		0	1	0	0	0	1
Autistic traits/risk	6	0				2			0	
ADHD symptoms/risk	5	1	0		1	0			0	
Additional Education Need	2	0				0				
Parent-child relationship	1	0	0							

Fig. 7.3 Neurodevelopmental disorders relating to ASMs. Numbers of studies reported are showed in the figure

lead to many different conclusions, such as multiple exposures to VPA or intraperitoneal injection and subcutaneous injection during organ formation mainly causing neural tube defects, while continuous exposure to VPA via microinfusion pump usually leads to decreased fetal weight and stillbirth, causing only a small number of neural tube defects at higher doses. Therefore, the conclusions of animal experiments need to be carefully discussed.

Up to now, the teratogenic animal experiments of ASMs have mainly focused on several traditional ASMs such as PHT, VPA, and CBZ (Table 7.2). The teratogenic effects of both VPA and PHT have been found in many different species, and there is a certain dose-dependency. The most common teratogenic patterns of VPA are skeletal malformations and neural tube defects, the former including axial bone malformations and accessory bone malformations, and the latter mainly involving incomplete closure of the forebrain neural tube. Different species and different strains of the same species show different sensitivities to teratogenic patterns and dose-response relationships, indicating that the teratogenic effects of VPA also need to consider genetic susceptibility. PHT-induced malformations are mainly of the cleft palate, with other malformations including various skeletal malformations, enlarged ventricles, renal malformations, cardiac malformations, ocular malformations, and other visceral malformations similar to those observed clinically in fetal hydantoin syndrome. Exposure to CBZ during organogenesis can slightly increase the incidence of cleft palate, enlarged ventricles, and growth retardation, while exposure to CBZ before and throughout pregnancy can significantly increase the incidence of central nervous system and genitourinary system defects, but overall, its use is still safer than that of VPA and PHT.

Research into the safety of VPA during pregnancy has also involved studies on the structure-teratogenicity relationship. VPA is a drug model that is very suitable for studying the relationship between chemical structure and teratogenic effects, and its teratogenicity depends on the combined action of the carboxyl group, C-2 hydrogen atom (α-COOH), and the C-2 branch (Sullivan and McElhatton 1975). Studies on the alkyl side chain of VPA have shown that when both alkyl side chains are aliphatic and contain three carbon atoms, the teratogenic potency is greatest, i.e., VPA (Fritz et al. 1976). Therefore, changes in the aforementioned three structures can affect its teratogenicity. Currently, studies have demonstrated this and found that amide derivatives of VPA and similar compounds, as well as urea derivatives of some structural isomers of VPA, have non-teratogenic effects or enantioselective teratogenic effects. Some of them also exhibit good antiepileptic activity, such as valproamide and valnoctamide.

7.3.3 Mechanisms of Teratogenicity

There is no consensus on the teratogenic mechanism of ASMs, and there are currently many hypotheses, mainly involving interference with folate metabolism, oxidative stress, effects on gene expression, and interference with ion channel function.

Table 7.2 Teratogenic animal experiments of antiseizure medications (Macdonald et al. 1989; Finnell et al. 1986, 1988; Spiegelstein et al. 2003; Okada et al. 2009; Lin et al. 2019; Turner et al. 1990; Eluma et al. 1984; Philbrook et al. 2019; Nau 1985, 1986a, b; Vorhees 1987; Binkerd et al. 1988; Ceylan et al. 2001; Petrere et al. 1986; Hendrickx et al. 1988; Lee et al. 2013; Sullivan and McElhatton 1977; Bennett et al. 1996; Jose et al. 2017; Vorhees et al. 1990; Sullivan and McElhatton 1975; Gibson and Becker 1968; Harbison and Becker 1969)

						Malformations				
ASMs	Animals	Exposure duration	Dosages	Teratogenic risk	Dose-dependence	Growth retardation	External malformations	Skeletal malformations	Internal organ malformations	Others
VPA	SWV mice	GD 8	~600 mg/kg	Teratogenic risk was higher in DBA/2 J and LM/Bc strain, and the skeletal abnormalities were more common than malformation in appearance and internal organ	Appearance malformations, visceral malformations, and skeletal malformations were dose-dependent		Orofacial clefts, neural tube defects (mainly anterior neural tube malformations)	Vertebral fusion/deformation, rib fusion, multiple ribs, increased vertebrae	Enlarged brain ventricles, renal pelvis dilation, uterine malformation in cornua uteri	GD 8:12 is the teratogenicity-sensitive period
	CD-1 mice	GD 8–16	~563 mg/kg	The incidence of neural tube defects is significantly higher than that of the control group (30% vs 1%)	The fetal weight decrease and the number of stillbirths exhibit a dose-dependent relationship	Decrease in fetal weight	Neural tube defect (particularly in the forebrain region), cleft palate	Microcephaly	Abnormalities in cardiac structure and a decrease in cardiac contractile function	
	NMRI mice	GD 6–9	~600 mg/kg	~63%	The decrease in fetal weight, stillbirth rate, and incidence of neural tube defects were dose-dependent	Decrease in fetal weight, fetal death	Neural tube defects			Minipumps administration primarily resulted in decreased fetal weight and fetal death, with high doses potentially leading to neural tube defects. Intermittent administration, subcutaneous injection, or intraperitoneal injection mainly induced neural tube defects

ASMs	Animals	Exposure duration	Dosages	Teratogenic risk	Dose-dependence	Malformations				Others
						Growth retardation	External malformations	Skeletal malformations	Internal organ malformations	
	DBA mice	GD 8	600 mg/kg	<SWV and LM/Bc			Neural tube defects			
	LM/Bc mice	GD 8	600 mg/kg	>DBA, <SWV			Neural tube defects			
	SD rats	GD 7–18	~600 mg/kg	~100%	Skeletal deformities and decreased fetal weight demonstrated a dose-dependent relationship		Neural tube malformations	The most common abnormalities observed are wavy ribs, followed by fused ribs, vertebral body absence or cleft, and curved/short/absent coccyx	The most common abnormalities observed are renal malformations, followed by cardiovascular abnormalities	
	Wistar rats	From 2 weeks before conception throughout the entire gestational period	~600 mg/kg	100% of cases induced vertebral arch malformation and neural tube defects in GAERS Wistar rats			Neural tube malformations (spina bifida predominate)			Embryonic morphological scores significantly decreased following in utero exposure to VPA, with notable occurrences of vertebral arch malformation and altered intervertebral spacing
	Dutch-belted rabbits	GD 6–18	~350 mg/kg	7–35%	Skeletal malformations exhibited a dose-dependent relationship			Vertebral, rib, and phalangeal malformation		

(continued)

Table 7.2 (continued)

ASMs	Animals	Exposure duration	Dosages	Teratogenic risk	Dose-dependence	Malformations				Others
						Growth retardation	External malformations	Skeletal malformations	Internal organ malformations	
	Rhesus monkeys	GD 21–50	~600 mg/kg	18/28	Dose-dependent toxicity manifested as intrauterine growth retardation, and skeletal malformations		Craniofacial malformations (round skull, frontal bossing, proptosis, low-set ears, flattened nasal angle, zygomatic arch abnormities, maxillary/ mandibular hypoplasia)	Axial skeletal malformations (vertebrae/ribs fused/ hypoplastic), appendicular skeletal malformations (long bones hypoplastic abnormal curvature, phalanges Aplastic/ hypoplastic)	Visceral malformations (ventricular septal defects and great vessel anomalies)	Craniofacial and skeletal malformations had a higher incidence compared with visceral malformations
	Zebrafish (wild-type AB strain)	5.25–72 hpf	6.25–100 mM	12–76%	With dose-dependent relationship	Growth retardation (12–94%)	Scoliosis (5%)			

ASMs	Animals	Exposure duration	Dosages	Teratogenic risk	Dose-dependence	Malformations				Others
						Growth retardation	External malformations	Skeletal malformations	Internal organ malformations	
CBZ	CD-1 mice	GD 8–16	~1664 mg/kg	~2.3%	The fetal weight decrease and the number of stillbirths exhibit a dose-dependent relationship		Cleft palate			
	SWV mice	From 2 weeks before conception throughout the entire gestational period	~1000 mg/kg	The teratogenic rate significantly increased compared to the controls				Skeletal abnormalities	Internal organ malformations were discovered	
	LM/Bc mice	From 2 weeks before conception throughout the entire gestational period	~2000 mg/kg	13.95–18.18%, but no significant statistical difference was observed compared to the controls	Without dose-dependent relationship				Cryptorchidism	
	BALB/c mice	GD 0	~600 mg/kg			Low birth weight and delayed physical development				
	SWR mice	From 2 weeks before conception throughout the entire gestational period	~2000 mg/kg	8.16–14.06% (no significant statistical difference was observed compared to the controls)	Without dose-dependent relationship				Enlarged brain ventricles, hydronephrosis	
	SD rats	GD 7–18	~600 mg/kg/day	2.3–21.7%	Skeletal abnormalities (delayed ossification centers) exhibit a dose-dependent relationship	Fetal weight reduced	Tail bending	Ribs absence	Edema, ventricular septal defect, omphalocele, hydronephrosis, umbilical hernia, esophageal dilation	
	Zebrafish (wild-type AB strain)	5.25–72 hpf	0.1–2 mM	31–100%	With dose-dependent relationship	Growth retardation (~100%)		Scoliosis (~11%), tail malformations (~8%)	Cardiac malformations (~44%)	

(continued)

Table 7.2 (continued)

ASMs	Animals	Exposure duration	Dosages	Teratogenic risk	Dose-dependence	Malformations				Others
						Growth retardation	External malformations	Skeletal malformations	Internal organ malformations	
PHT	CI mice	GD 6–16	~	0–11.1% (cleft palate)			Cleft palate			
	A/J mice	GD 7–13	~50 mg/kg	0–30.8%			Cleft palate with or without cleft lip			Exposure to PHT during the late stages of embryonic development can cause cleft palate with or without cleft lip
	SWR mice	GD 8–15	~150 mg/kg	0–15.2%	The rate of stillbirth, malformation, and growth retardation all show a dose-dependent relationship		Eye opening, orofacial malformations (cleft palate with or without cleft lip)	Hallux valgus, long bones were shortened	Hydronephrosis, hydrocephalus	Exposure during early pregnancy commonly results in eye opening, toe deviation, skeletal malformations, hydronephrosis, and hydrocephalus, while exposure during late pregnancy is more commonly associated with orofacial malformations
	NMRI mice	GD 6–15	~170 mg/kg	0.3–9.3% (Cleft palate)	With dose-dependent relationship		Cleft palate			
	SWV mice	From 2 weeks before conception throughout the entire gestational period	~60 mg/kg	41–85%	With dose-dependent relationship	Fetal weight reduction		Hypoplasia of the phalanx	Brian ventricular dilation/ hypoplasia, ventricular septal defect hydronephrosis	

ASMs	Animals	Exposure duration	Dosages	Teratogenic risk	Dose-dependence	Malformations				Others
						Growth retardation	External malformations	Skeletal malformations	Internal organ malformations	
	CD-1mice	GD 6–16	~90 mg/kg	~75.8% (Amicarelli et al. 2000)	With dose-dependent relationship		(Complete) cleft palate	Curved coccyx, delayed ossification of the foot bones, sternal defects/ fusion/cleft	Cryptorchidism, ovarian ectopia	
	LM/Bc mice	From 2 weeks before conception throughout the entire gestational period	~60 mg/kg	40–56%	With dose-dependent relationship	Fetal weight reduction		Hypoplasia of the phalanx	Cerebral ventricular dilatation/ hypoplasia, ventricular septal defect, hydronephrosis	
	C57mice	From 15 days before conception throughout the entire gestational period	~60 mg/kg	29–77%			Ocular anophthalmia, microphthalmia, cleft lip	Hypoplasia of the phalanx, missing or misaligned sternabrae, delayed ossification and hypoplastic growth of the facial bones	Ventricular septal defects of the heart, hypoplastic atria, transposition of the great vessels, hypoplastic kidney, hydronephrosis, dilated or immaturely developed cerebral ventricles of the brain	The occurrence of these defects was correlated with maternal serum concentrations, but not with the maternal seizure disorder

(continued)

Table 7.2 (continued)

ASMs	Animals	Exposure duration	Dosages	Teratogenic risk	Dose-dependence	Malformations				Others
						Growth retardation	External malformations	Skeletal malformations	Internal organ malformations	
PB	SD rats	GD 7–15	~200 mg/kg	~54%	With dose-dependent relationship	Growth retardation	Cleft palate		Hydronephrosis, uterine malformation	Exposure during early pregnancy commonly results in hydronephrosis and uterine malformation, while exposure during late pregnancy is more commonly associated with cleft palate
	Cats	GD 10–22	~2 mg/kg	1/19–4/38	With dose-dependent relationship		Cleft palate	Rigid wrists, limb malformations, missing digits	Umbilical hernia	
	SWV mice	From 3 weeks before conception throughout the entire gestational period	~240 mg/kg	15.4–37.5%			Cleft palate	Delayed ossification is most common, with others including digit abnormalities, sternal malformations, abnormal vertebral body centers, craniofacial deformities, and occipital bone deformities	Neurological malformations, dilatation/ hypoplasia, cryptorchidism, ventricular septal defect, and left heart hypoplasia	Skeletal malformations are the most common, followed by neurological and renal malformations

ASMs	Animals	Exposure duration	Dosages	Teratogenic risk	Dose-dependence	Malformations				Others
						Growth retardation	External malformations	Skeletal malformations	Internal organ malformations	
	C57 mice	From 3 weeks before conception throughout the entire gestational period	~240 mg/kg	14.3–28.6%				Delayed ossification is most common, with others including digit abnormalities, sternal malformations, abnormal vertebral body centers, craniofacial deformities, and occipital bone deformities	Neurological malformations, dilatation/ hypoplasia, cryptorchidism, ventricular septal defect, and left heart hypoplasia	Skeletal malformations are the most common, followed by neurological and renal malformations
	LM/Bc mice	From 3 weeks before conception throughout the entire gestational period	~240 mg/kg	22.1–46.7%	Skeletal and cardiac malformations showed a dose-dependent relationship		Cleft palate	Delayed ossification is most common, with others including digit abnormalities, sternal malformations, abnormal vertebral body centers, craniofacial deformities, and occipital bone deformities	Neurological malformations, dilatation/ hypoplasia, cryptorchidism, ventricular septal defect, and left heart hypoplasia	Skeletal malformations are the most common, followed by neurological and renal malformations
	CD-1mice	GD 6–16	~60 mg/kg	~2.4%	With dose-dependent relationship		Complete cleft palate			
CLN	CD-1mice	GD 6–16	~1.8 mg/kg	~4.3%	With dose-dependent relationship		Complete cleft palate			
LTG	Zebrafish (wild-type AB strain)	5.25–72 hpf	0.05–1 mM	0–65%	With dose-dependent relationship	Growth retardation (~25%)	Scoliosis (~35%), head malformations (~5%)	Tail malformations (~11%)	Cardiac malformations (~40%), yolk sac malformations (~30%)	

(continued)

Table 7.2 (continued)

ASMs	Animals	Exposure duration	Dosages	Teratogenic risk	Dose-dependence	Malformations					Others
						Growth retardation	External malformations	Skeletal malformations	Internal organ malformations		
LEV	SWV/Fnn mice	GD 8–12	~2000 mg/kg	29–49% (skeletal malformations)				Hypoplasia of the phalanx			No specific malformations were found to be associated
	Zebrafish (wild-type AB strain)	5.25–72 hpf	1–100 mM	0–13%		Growth retardation (~13%)			Cardiac malformations (~13%)		
TPM	Rats	–	–	–				Partial or complete fingers missing			
	Rabbits	–	–	–				Rib and vertebral malformations			
	Zebrafish (wild-type AB strain)	5.25–72 hpf	~50 mM	25–100%	The dose-dependent relationship is not clear, but malformations were observed at each dose level	Growth retardation (~50%)	Scoliosis (~50%)	Tail malforma-tions(~8%)	Cardiac malformations (~100%), yolk sac malformations (~100%)		
OXC	SWV/Fnn mice	From 2 weeks before conception throughout the entire gestational period	~1000 mg/kg	2–11% (0–18% skeletal malformations, 4–7% internal organ malformations)				Skeletal malformations	Internal organ malformations		
	Rats	–	~300 mg/kg(OXC) ~500 mg/kg(MHD)	With teratogenic effects							
GBP	ICR mice	GD 1–6, 7–12, 13–17	~452 mg/kg	Malformations were observed in the mid-gestation treated groups	The dose-dependent relationship is not clear, but malformations were observed at each dose level	Growth retardation	Orofacial malformations, open eyes, cataracts, short thick neck	Limb dysplasia			

ASMs	Animals	Exposure duration	Dosages	Teratogenic risk	Dose-dependence	Malformations				Others
						Growth retardation	External malformations	Skeletal malformations	Internal organ malformations	
ZNS	Mice	During pregnancy	~200 mg/kg							250 mg/kg exhibited maternal and fetal toxicity, while 500 mg/kg demonstrated teratogenicity
	Rats	During pregnancy	~500 mg/kg		With dose-dependent relationship	Low birth weight		Delayed ossification	Cardiac malformation (ventricular septal defect)	
	Dogs	GD 14–35	~60 mg/kg		>30 mg/kg demonstrated teratogenicity			Coccygeal fusion/ malformations, lumbar vertebral malformations	Cardiac malformations, spleen and thymic hypoplasia, umbilical hernia	
	Machin	GD 21–45	~20 mg/kg		10 mg/kg exhibited maternal toxicity and fetal death					
PGB	Wistar rats	GD 6–17	~2500 mg/kg	0.4–1.1%						No teratogenic pattern related to drug treatment was observed
	Albino mice	GD 6–15	~2500 mg/kg							No teratogenic pattern related to drug treatment was observed
	New Zealand white rabbits	GD 6–20	~1250 mg/kg							No teratogenic pattern related to drug treatment was observed

(continued)

Table 7.2 (continued)

ASMs	Animals	Exposure duration	Dosages	Teratogenic risk	Dose-dependence	Malformations					Others
						Growth retardation	External malformations	Skeletal malformations	Internal organ malformations		
LCM	Mice	Two days before mating and until the 14th day post-coitus	~120 mg/kg	4.3–12.2%, significantly higher than controls			Neural tube defects, facial malformations		Cardiovascular malformations		
	Zebrafish (wild-type AB strain)	5.25–72 hpf	0.5–10 mm	10–100%	With dose-dependent relationship	Growth retardation (~100%)	Scoliosis(~33%)	Tail malformations (~17%)	Cardiac malformations (~58%)		
VGB	New Zealand white rabbits	–	–	–			Cleft palate				

VPA valproate, *CBZ* carbamazepine, *PHT* phenytoin, *PB* phenobarbital, *CLN* clonazepam, *LTG* lamotrigine, *LEV* levetiracetam, *TPM* topiramate, *OXC* oxcarbazepine, *GBP* gabapentin, *ZNS* zonisamide, *PGB* pregabalin, *LCM* lacosamide, *VGB* vigabatrin

The teratogenic mechanism of VPA mainly involves the following aspects: (1) Interference with folate metabolism. VPA can reduce placental folate levels, and its mechanism may involve non-competitive inhibition of folate receptors by VPA and interference with MTHFR. (2) Effects on gene expression. VPA can inhibit histone deacetylases (HDACs), which can affect the expression of many downstream genes, including zinc finger transcription factors, hypoxia, p53, and cyclins. This can lead to cell cycle arrest, homologous gene silencing, cell growth arrest, and death, disrupting neurodevelopment and skeletal development, leading to malformations. VPA and its teratogenic analogs can also activate PPARδ (a nuclear receptor that regulates gene expression and cell growth), suggesting that PPARδ may be involved in the teratogenic mechanism of VPA. (3) Oxidative stress and DNA damage. In vitro studies have shown that VPA can increase the formation of reactive oxygen species (ROS) and inhibit the differentiation of myocardial cells, and these changes can be counteracted by pretreatment with antioxidants. In vivo studies have also found that hydrogen peroxide can prevent birth defects caused by VPA. Since no changes in markers of oxidative damage were observed with VPA exposure, VPA is more likely to mediate the occurrence of malformations through its effects on redox-sensitive signaling pathways.

The teratogenic mechanism of PHT is similar to that of VPA: (1) Induction of CYP450, increasing folate metabolism. (2) Causing fetal hypoxia. PHT can inhibit the HERG channel, which is responsible for the rapid activation of the delayed rectifier potassium current (IKr). Animal experiments have shown that normal embryonic heart function depends on the IKr current in the early embryo, and inhibition of IKr can cause bradycardia and arrhythmia, leading to fetal hypoxia, which is related to the limb defects, cardiac malformations, cleft lip, and midfacial hypoplasia caused by PHT, especially limb defects. (3) Oxidative stress caused by drug active metabolites. PHT is converted to active intermediates by CYP2C9 in the liver, leading to oxidative stress that can damage cellular macromolecules such as DNA, proteins, and lipids, and can alter normal signaling pathways by activating redox-sensitive transcription factors. Moreover, the expression levels of superoxide dismutase, catalase, and glutathione peroxidase in the early embryonic development process are lower than those in the maternal body, making them more susceptible to oxidative damage from ROS. Microsomal epoxide hydrolase (EPHX1) can metabolize PHT active intermediates into inactive compounds. Population-based studies have shown that EPHX1 Y113/H139 has a protective effect on craniofacial malformations after PHT exposure, while EPHX1 H113/R139 may increase the risk of craniofacial malformations after PHT exposure; in vivo studies suggest that the latter has lower metabolic capacity than the former.

Apart from VPA and PHT, CBZ, PB, and PRM are all associated with folate deficiency, and LTG can also interfere with folate metabolism by inhibiting dihydrofolate reductase. Folate deficiency has been shown to be one of the important causes of fetal neural tube defects, and some researchers have found that abnormal folate metabolism is a risk factor for congenital heart disease and cleft lip/palate. While folate supplementation has been shown to reduce the incidence of neural tube defects in the general population, its effect in women with epilepsy is still under investigation. Current research indicates that perinatal folate supplementation may not reduce the incidence of congenital malformations in offspring and may also fail to reduce VPA-induced neural tube defects and embryonic toxicity.

GBP and PGB are gamma-aminobutyric acid analogs with high affinity for the α2d subunit of calcium channels in the brain, spinal cord, skeletal muscle, and cardiac muscle, especially the α2d-1 and 2d-2 subtypes. The α2d-1 subtype plays a key role in the adhesion and migration of myoblasts, which can affect the development of muscle and nerve tissues. This may explain the cardiac developmental defects caused by early pregnancy exposure to GBP and PGB.

Overall, current clinical research suggests that ASMs are associated with certain relatively specific congenital malformations, such as cleft lip/palate, neural tube defects, cardiac malformations, and genitourinary system defects, all of which can be attributed to abnormalities in the embryonic folding and fusion process. Therefore, there is a hypothesis that interference with ion channel function by ASMs can disrupt the balance of resting potentials that provide positional or other growth and developmental information for cells and tissues during embryonic development, and even affect downstream gene expression, thereby influencing processes such as the left-right patterning of heart development, neuronal development, and eye development.

7.4 Postpartum Counseling for Women with Epilepsy

Ziyi Chen

Due to the change in life roles after childbirth, the decline of attention, and the change of physiological conditions, WWE bear a large mental and psychological pressure. As a result, postnatal counseling is critical for WWE. In WWE, changes in blood drug concentration after delivery should be monitored closely, with dosages adjusted according to blood drug concentrations in order to prevent risks caused by excessive drug concentrations. In addition, it is also crucial for WWE to maintain their physical and mental health after delivery. Patients and their families should pay attention to the emotional changes of patients in a timely manner to prevent the occurrence of postpartum anxiety, depression, and other mental diseases. During postpartum counseling, WWE should be informed of the benefits and risks of breastfeeding and encourage patients to breastfeed, but should also be concerned about the occurrence of adverse fetal reactions during the feeding process. During breastfeeding, WWE need to understand feeding precautions, avoid fatigue, and ensure sufficient rest while ensuring efficient feeding, so as to avoid inducing epilepsy.

References

Amicarelli F, Tiboni GM, Colafarina S, et al. Antioxidant and GSH-related enzyme response to a single teratogenic exposure to the anticonvulsant phenytoin: temporospatial evaluation. Teratology. 2000;62(2):100–7.

Bennett GD, Amore BM, Finnell RH, et al. Teratogenicity of carbamazepine-10, 11-epoxide and oxcarbazepine in the SWV mouse. J Pharmacol Exp Ther. 1996;279(3):1237–42.

Bennett HA, Einarson A, Taddio A, Koren G, Einarson TR. Prevalence of depression during pregnancy: systematic review. Obstet Gynecol. 2004;103(4):698–709.

Binkerd PE, Rowland JM, Nau H, et al. Evaluation of valproic acid (VPA) developmental toxicity and pharmacokinetics in Sprague-Dawley rats. Fundam Appl Toxicol. 1988;11(3):485–93.
Bjork MH, Veiby G, Reiter SC, Berle JO, Daltveit AK, Spigset O, et al. Depression and anxiety in women with epilepsy during pregnancy and after delivery: a prospective population-based cohort study on frequency, risk factors, medication, and prognosis. Epilepsia. 2015;56(1):28–39.
Ceylan S, Duru S, Ceylan S. Valproic acid sodium-induced spina bifida occulta in the rat. Neurosurg Rev. 2001;24(1):31–4.
Eluma FO, Sucheston ME, Hayes TG, et al. Teratogenic effects of dosage levels and time of administration of carbamazepine, sodium valproate, and diphenylhydantoin on craniofacial development in the CD-1 mouse fetus. J Craniofac Genet Dev Biol. 1984;4(3):191–210.
Finnell RH, Mohl VK, Bennett GD, et al. Failure of epoxide formation to influence carbamazepine-induced teratogenesis in a mouse model. Teratog Carcinog Mutagen. 1986;6(5):393–401.
Finnell RH, Bennett GD, Karras SB, et al. Common hierarchies of susceptibility to the induction of neural tube defects in mouse embryos by valproic acid and its 4-propyl-4-pentenoic acid metabolite. Teratology. 1988;38(4):313–20.
Fritz H, Muller D, Hess R. Comparative study of the teratogenicity of phenobarbitone, diphenylhydantoin and carbamazepine in mice. Toxicology. 1976;6(3):323–30.
Galanti M, Newport DJ, Pennell PB, Titchner D, Newman M, Knight BT, et al. Postpartum depression in women with epilepsy: influence of antiepileptic drugs in a prospective study. Epilepsy Behav. 2009;16(3):426–30.
Gavin NI, Gaynes BN, Lohr KN, Meltzer-Brody S, Gartlehner G, Swinson T. Perinatal depression: a systematic review of prevalence and incidence. Obstet Gynecol. 2005;106(5 Pt 1):1071–83.
Gibson JE, Becker BA. Teratogenic effects of diphenylhydantoin in Swiss-Webster and A-J mice. Proc Soc Exp Biol Med. 1968;128(3):905–9.
Harbison RD, Becker BA. Relation of dosage and time of administration of diphenylhydantoin to its teratogenic effect in mice. Teratology. 1969;2(4):305–11.
Hendrickx AG, Nau H, Binkerd P, et al. Valproic acid developmental toxicity and pharmacokinetics in the rhesus monkey: an interspecies comparison. Teratology. 1988;38(4):329–45.
Jose M, Sreelatha HV, James MV, et al. Teratogenic effects of carbamazepine in mice. Ann Indian Acad Neurol. 2017;20(2):132–7.
Lee SH, Kang JW, Lin T, et al. Teratogenic potential of antiepileptic drugs in the zebrafish model. Biomed Res Int. 2013;2013:726478.
Lin JJ, Mula M, Hermann BP. Uncovering the neurobehavioural comorbidities of epilepsy over the lifespan. Lancet. 2012;380(9848):1180–92.
Lin YL, Bialer M, Cabrera RM, et al. Teratogenicity of valproic acid and its constitutional isomer, amide derivative valnoctamide in mice. Birth Defects Res. 2019;111(14):1013–23.
Macdonald KB, Juriloff DM, Harris MJ. Developmental study of neural tube closure in a mouse stock with a high incidence of exencephaly. Teratology. 1989;39(2):195–213.
Nau H. Teratogenic valproic acid concentrations: infusion by implanted minipumps vs conventional injection regimen in the mouse. Toxicol Appl Pharmacol. 1985;80(2):243–50.
Nau H. Valproic acid teratogenicity in mice after various administration and phenobarbital-pretreatment regimens: the parent drug and not one of the metabolites assayed is implicated as teratogen. Fundam Appl Toxicol. 1986a;6(4):662–8.
Nau H. Transfer of valproic acid and its main active unsaturated metabolite to the gestational tissue: correlation with neural tube defect formation in the mouse. Teratology. 1986b;33(1):21–7.
Okada A, Noyori H, Yagen B, et al. Anticonvulsant profile and teratogenic evaluation of potent new analogues of a valproic acid urea derivative in NMRI mice. Birth Defects Res B Dev Reprod Toxicol. 2009;86(5):394–401.
Petrere JA, Anderson JA, Sakowski R, et al. Teratogenesis of calcium valproate in rabbits. Teratology. 1986;34(3):263–9.
Philbrook NA, Nikolovska A, Maciver RD, et al. Characterizing the effects of in utero exposure to valproic acid on murine fetal heart development. Birth Defects Res. 2019;111(19):1551–60.
Quiske A, Helmstaedter C, Lux S, Elger CE. Depression in patients with temporal lobe epilepsy is related to mesial temporal sclerosis. Epilepsy Res. 2000;39(2):121–5.

Rai D, Kerr MP, McManus S, Jordanova V, Lewis G, Brugha TS. Epilepsy and psychiatric comorbidity: a nationally representative population-based study. Epilepsia. 2012;53(6):1095–103.
Reiter SF, Veiby G, Daltveit AK, Engelsen BA, Gilhus NE. Psychiatric comorbidity and social aspects in pregnant women with epilepsy—the Norwegian Mother and Child Cohort Study. Epilepsy Behav. 2013;29(2):379–85.
Spiegelstein O, Chatterjie N, Alexander G, et al. Teratogenicity of valproate conjugates with anticonvulsant activity in mice. Epilepsy Res. 2003;57(2–3):145–52.
Sullivan FM, McElhatton PR. Teratogenic activity of the antiepileptic drugs phenobarbital, phenytoin, and primidone in mice. Toxicol Appl Pharmacol. 1975;34(2):271–82.
Sullivan FM, McElhatton PR. A comparison of the teratogenic activity of the antiepileptic drugs carbamazepine, clonazepam, ethosuximide, phenobarbital, phenytoin, and primidone in mice. Toxicol Appl Pharmacol. 1977;40(2):365–78.
Turner S, Sucheston ME, De Philip RM, et al. Teratogenic effects on the neuroepithelium of the CD-1 mouse embryo exposed in utero to sodium valproate. Teratology. 1990;41(4):421–42.
Turner K, Piazzini A, Franza A, Fumarola C, Chifari R, Marconi AM, et al. Postpartum depression in women with epilepsy versus women without epilepsy. Epilepsy Behav. 2006;9(2):293–7.
Turner K, Piazzini A, Franza A, Marconi AM, Canger R, Canevini MP. Epilepsy and postpartum depression. Epilepsia. 2009;50(Suppl 1):24–7.
Vorhees CV. Teratogenicity and developmental toxicity of valproic acid in rats. Teratology. 1987;35(2):195–202.
Vorhees CV, Acuff KD, Weisenburger WP, et al. Teratogenicity of carbamazepine in rats. Teratology. 1990;41(3):311–7.

Suggested Readings

Agency EM. Zonegran. https://www.ema.europa.eu/en/medicines/human/EPAR/zonegran.
Azzato EM, Chen RA, Wacholder S, et al. Maternal EPHX1 polymorphisms and risk of phenytoin-induced congenital malformations. Pharmacogenet Genomics. 2010;20(1):58–63.
Barker LC, Dennis CL, Hussain-Shamsy N, Stewart DE, Grigoriadis S, Metcalfe K, et al. Decision-making about antidepressant medication use in pregnancy: a comparison between women making the decision in the preconception period versus in pregnancy. BMC Psychiatry. 2020;20(1):54.
Beyenburg S, Mitchell AJ, Schmidt D, Elger CE, Reuber M. Anxiety in patients with epilepsy: systematic review and suggestions for clinical management. Epilepsy Behav. 2005;7(2):161–71.
Bodeker K, Fuchs A, Fuhrer D, Kluczniok D, Dittrich K, Reichl C, et al. Impact of maternal early life maltreatment and maternal history of depression on child psychopathology: mediating role of maternal sensitivity? Child Psychiatry Hum Dev. 2019;50(2):278–90.
Costa R, Magalhaes LM, Graca J, et al. Eslicarbazepine acetate exposure in pregnant women with epilepsy. Seizure. 2018;58:72–4.
Crawford P. Best practice guidelines for the management of women with epilepsy. Epilepsia. 2005;46(Suppl 9):117–24.
Dansky LV, Rosenblatt DS, Andermann E. Mechanisms of teratogenesis: folic acid and antiepileptic therapy. Neurology. 1992;42(4 Suppl 5):32–42.
Fathe K, Palacios A, Finnell RH. Brief report novel mechanism for valproate-induced teratogenicity. Birth Defects Res A Clin Mol Teratol. 2014;100(8):592–7.
Finegersh A, Avedissian C, Shamim S, Dustin I, Thompson PM, Theodore WH. Bilateral hippocampal atrophy in temporal lobe epilepsy: effect of depressive symptoms and febrile seizures. Epilepsia. 2011;52(4):689–97.
Finnell RH. Phenytoin-induced teratogenesis: a mouse model. Science. 1981;211(4481):483–4.
Finnell RH, Chernoff GF. Mouse fetal hydantoin syndrome: effects of maternal seizures. Epilepsia. 1982;23(4):423–9.
Finnell RH, Shields HE, Taylor SM, et al. Strain differences in phenobarbital-induced teratogenesis in mice. Teratology. 1987a;35(2):177–85.

Finnell RH, Shields HE, Chernoff GF. Variable patterns in anticonvulsant drug-induced malformations in mice: comparisons of phenytoin and phenobarbital. Teratog Carcinog Mutagen. 1987b;7(6):541–9.
Glauser TA. Topiramate. Epilepsia. 1999;40(Suppl 5):S71–80.
Harbison RD, Becker BA. Diphenylhydantoin teratogenicity in rats. Toxicol Appl Pharmacol. 1972;22(2):193–200.
Isoherranen N, Spiegelstein O, Bialer M, et al. Developmental outcome of levetiracetam, its major metabolite in humans, 2-pyrrolidinone N-butyric acid, and its enantiomer (R)-alpha-ethyl-oxo-pyrrolidine acetamide in a mouse model of teratogenicity. Epilepsia. 2003;44(10):1280–8.
Karabiber H, Sonmezgoz E, Ozerol E, et al. Effects of valproate and carbamazepine on serum levels of homocysteine, vitamin B12, and folic acid. Brain Dev. 2003;25(2):113–5.
Khera KS. A teratogenicity study on hydroxyurea and diphenylhydantoin in cats. Teratology. 1979;20(3):447–52.
Kothari A, de Laat J, Dulhunty JM, Bruxner G. Perceptions of pregnant women regarding antidepressant and anxiolytic medication use during pregnancy. Australas Psychiatry. 2019;27(2):117–20.
Lampen A, Carlberg C, Nau H. Peroxisome proliferator-activated receptor delta is a specific sensor for teratogenic valproic acid derivatives. Eur J Pharmacol. 2001;431(1):25–33.
Lopez-Escobar B, Fernandez-Torres R, Vargas-Lopez V, et al. Lacosamide intake during pregnancy increases the incidence of foetal malformations and symptoms associated with schizophrenia in the offspring of mice. Sci Rep. 2020;10(1):7615.
McDevitt JM, Gautieri RF, Mann DE Jr. Comparative teratogenicity of cortisone and phenytoin in mice. J Pharm Sci. 1981;70(6):631–4.
Mehndiratta P, Sajatovic M. Treatments for patients with comorbid epilepsy and depression: a systematic literature review. Epilepsy Behav. 2013;28(1):36–40.
Morse DC. Embryo-fetal developmental toxicity studies with pregabalin in mice and rabbits. Birth Defects Res B Dev Reprod Toxicol. 2016;107(2):85–93.
Morse DC, Henck JW, Bailey SA. Developmental toxicity studies with pregabalin in rats: significance of alterations in skull bone morphology. Birth Defects Res B Dev Reprod Toxicol. 2016;107(2):94–107.
Mula M, Monaco F, Trimble MR. Use of psychotropic drugs in patients with epilepsy: interactions and seizure risk. Expert Rev Neurother. 2004;4(6):953–64.
Munk-Olsen T, Laursen TM, Pedersen CB, Mors O, Mortensen PB. New parents and mental disorders: a population-based register study. JAMA. 2006;296(21):2582–9.
Na L, Wartenberg M, Nau H, et al. Anticonvulsant valproic acid inhibits cardiomyocyte differentiation of embryonic stem cells by increasing intracellular levels of reactive oxygen species. Birth Defects Res A Clin Mol Teratol. 2003;67(3):174–80.
Okada A, Fujiwara M. Molecular approaches to developmental malformations using analogous forms of valproic acid. Congenit Anom (Kyoto). 2006;46(2):68–75.
Paulson RB, Paulson GW, Jreissaty S. Phenytoin and carbamazepine in production of cleft palates in mice. Comparison of teratogenic effects. Arch Neurol. 1979;36(13):832–6.
Prakash, Prabhu LV, Rai R, et al. Teratogenic effects of the anticonvulsant gabapentin in mice. Singapore Med J. 2008;49(1):47–53.
Priel A, Djalovski A, Zagoory-Sharon O, Feldman R. Maternal depression impacts child psychopathology across the first decade of life: oxytocin and synchrony as markers of resilience. J Child Psychol Psychiatry. 2019;60(1):30–42.
Rubinchik-Stern M, Shmuel M, Bar J, et al. Adverse placental effects of valproic acid: studies in perfused human placentas. Epilepsia. 2018;59(5):993–1003.
Tecoma ES. Oxcarbazepine. Epilepsia. 1999;40(Suppl 5):S37–46.
Tung EW, Winn LM. Valproic acid increases formation of reactive oxygen species and induces apoptosis in postimplantation embryos: a role for oxidative stress in valproic acid-induced neural tube defects. Mol Pharmacol. 2011;80(6):979–87.
Vazquez B, Tomson T, Dobrinsky C, et al. Perampanel and pregnancy. Epilepsia. 2021;62(3):698–708.

Webster WS, Abela D. The effect of hypoxia in development. Birth Defects Res C Embryo Today. 2007;81(3):215–28.

Wegner C, Nau H. Alteration of embryonic folate metabolism by valproic acid during organogenesis: implications for mechanism of teratogenesis. Neurology. 1992;42(4 Suppl 5):17–24.

Winterfeld U, Merlob P, Baud D, et al. Pregnancy outcome following maternal exposure to pregabalin may call for concern. Neurology. 2016;86(24):2251–7.

Woody CA, Ferrari AJ, Siskind DJ, Whiteford HA, Harris MG. A systematic review and meta-regression of the prevalence and incidence of perinatal depression. J Affect Disord. 2017;219:86–92.

Xu A, Wang W, Jiang X. The roles of MTRR and MTHFR gene polymorphisms in congenital heart diseases: a meta-analysis. Biosci Rep. 2018;38(6):BSR20181160.

Zahn CA, Morrell MJ, Collins SD, et al. Management issues for women with epilepsy: a review of the literature. Neurology. 1998;51(4):949–56.